making meant to be

ONE WOMAN'S JOURNEY WITH SECONDARY INFERTILITY

Tracy McKay

Copyright 2012 Tracy McKay
All rights reserved.

to Chad

acknowledgements

I would like to thank Michael S, Paulina J, Ashley W, and Judy W for mentorship, design assistance, and technical advice. Thanks to Trace, Lis, and Peeps for inspiration and sisterhood. And thanks to Mom, Jim, Dad, and Sue for support, insight, and love.

I have changed most names of the people I have included in this story.

making meant to be

I

i have a picture of my brother and me when I am maybe five and he is seven-and-a-half. It is a faded picture and our bare skin glows white as we sit on a log in the middle of a river with nothing but shorts on. Our legs dangle in the freckled water; our heads tip in two directions; my brother is holding a half-eaten roll of crackers in his right hand. I don't know how long we were out there, the sun on our sides, straddling the fallen tree smooth and gone white, too. I don't know what we were saying, if we were saying anything at all.

I used to look at that picture and try to remember what it was like to be that girl, try to feel the water, the sun, the simple pull of my brother being there next to me.

But now I look and think of my mom, think of the sand or grass or maybe rock beneath her shoes as she stood on the riverbank looking at her two kids and their two bodies so easy in their skins. Surely she can't hear them with the river running and their heads turned, but she is them and she is not them as she holds the cool of the camera and brings it to her nose.

Life will go in this quiet tumble, teaching and learning, giving and taking, each kid with their differences and their sameness and her knowing it's possible to love this way twice.

At night she will listen through the bedroom wall to what it is between them: their chatter, their giggles, their silence. She will feel complete.

She finds the metal o with her index finger.

The camera clicks.

Two. It has always been two.

I don't know when or how desire starts (was I already feeling it out on that log?), but when people would ask, it was easy to answer. Even when I'd play the game MASH with a girl in the fourth or fifth grade (whenever it is that you start having enough crushes to list five initials down the edge of the page and can name five places that aren't stores or classrooms or friends' houses), I'd never be afraid when my forecast ended up being that I'd have sixteen kids. I may have been a little quaky if the administrator of the game, the girl pushing the pencil line to a spiral had said, "No, you have to put someone you don't like!" in that small-girl bossiness, and I had put EB and actually had to endure the bossiness turned guffaw as pigtails bounced and no hand thought to cover those two buck-teeth going topside. "Tracy's going to marry Earl! Ha, ha, ha!"

It would be that, that statement that would later leave me wondering, as I'd turn to see fat-faced Earl-the-Crotch-Pincher googling his eyes everywhere but at the book in front of him during silent reading, if it was actually possible. Could I end up with him? The likelihood of this scared me, as if I had no say in it, or as if one day I might actually blip into a girl who would want to hug and I guess kiss someone who put his hand on girls' bottoms in the lunch line and didn't read during silent reading and whose best friend had warts on his thumbs. Could I just change? So my preferences or my understanding of how one ends up in some big white dress saying, "I do" was beyond me, something I'd have to go learn. But the kids thing? I had that one covered. I was sure. Even when pigtail-mouth would be squawking about the sixteen kids we were going to have in a shack in Mississippi, I didn't worry. Two kids. One boy and one girl. Ol' Earl would just have to outsource if he wanted the other fourteen.

Maybe this kind of desire, something that has been there so long it doesn't even seem to have a beginning, is not desire but expectation. Because having two kids is not something I only want; it's just what's meant to be.

I am thirty-seven. My daughter just turned three.

We moved two months ago and there are still boxes all over the house. I wake up and lie still and wait for my husband Chad to be out of the bathroom. He's all splishes and splashes and taps and gargles, and inevitably, just when it goes quiet and I think he's about to exit, his razor snaps to a buzz.

I can see him in there without seeing him: bare-chested and bent with his ropy arm straight as his long fingers halfheartedly drape over the edge of the sink.

He clears his throat with that wha-too kind of sound that's right from the How-to-Hock-a-Good-Loogie cue card and reminds me of me and my brother in the back of the Spruce Street house. We were spitting in the dirt by the laundry line and he was saying, "No, end over end. A loogie goes end over end." He had done his fingers how you do when you're winding dental floss.

"Like a helicopter?" I had said.

"Yeah. But on its side," he had said.

Chad's still running the water. It rushes in the bathroom like a wide-mouthed river. Like Niagara Falls.

I have to pee. I've actually been having to pee for what seems like four dreams ago when I was running on a sidewalk looking for a place to pee. Somehow I had forced sleep and made it to this point, but now I feel like I will burst. My ovulation predictor sticks are in the master bathroom, and although I'd love to just use a different bathroom and test later, the first urine of the morning is the most concentrated and therefore the most definitive for the tests that matter right now: ovulation predicting and pregnancy.

I had once used late-in-the-day urine for a pregnancy test about a year-and-a-half ago. I hadn't been drinking a lot, but I still doubted the results when there was only one pink line. Maybe it was bad lighting. I held the test to the window. One line. Maybe I had the results window and the control window reversed and it's still processing.

I checked the box. Nope, the square is the control, the oval the results. Oh! It hit me then. I didn't use morning pee!

Happy to have regained my hope, I drove to the store to buy another test. I only bought the box with a single test because those were the days when I still thought, why pay more for two since if you are pregnant, you will be stuck with a test you will never use.

I had spent the rest of the day willing myself to wait until the next morning to test again. But I haven't had anything to drink in four hours, I'd pitch to myself. No, morning pee, you idiot! would counter that one voice who sounded a lot like Mr. T from *The A-Team*. It bothered me that I could be channeling a voice with that much testosterone (could Mr. T be throwing my hormones out of whack?), but obedience was worth more than fear. Be good. Do what the man says. You will be rewarded. Because somehow, somewhere, that kind of thing (the discipline, the self-restraint, anything that requires discomfort or a reigning in of habitual abundance) must matter. In the cosmos it must mean something because by telling myself no, I'm sending the message to whoever is listening that I am doing my part.

But the next morning? There had still only been one line. Not pregnant. Again.

Chad blows his nose, or does something that sounds like large plosive exhales through a nostril without having anything to catch it on the other end. Is this a joke? Is there an audition going on in there? Doesn't he know I have to pee?

But he doesn't. Or he does, but he doesn't know why

this pee is so important. I haven't told him that after two-and-a-half years of doing nothing, using sticks, charting, trying to "just relax," I am back to using the sticks again as a final push to seal the deal. Helena is three. Tack on the ten months gestational period and we are approaching the four-year age gap Chad and I had originally agreed was the limit. Four years between siblings was already challenging all the things I pictured them doing together: shoving action figures in the dehumidifier, singing in the backseat, walking to campground bathrooms kicking rocks, yelling and saying horrible things but passing each other at school the next day and still loving that familiar face, the face that would be there long after Chad and I were gone.

I roll to my side. He's got to be out soon.

Helena's doorknob rattles. There is a rub of wood and a suck of air. She must be standing there, standing at the small gate we have extended in her door.

"Mama, where are you? Mama, where are you?" she sings.

The water in the bathroom goes off. On. Off.

I want to yell, "Chad, you're on duty!", but I don't want to make noise. The light in our bedroom is like the ocean; it reminds me of the early morning when the fog is thick and shapes are dim. I lie still and want to stay like this, half my face feeling underwater, watching, waiting.

Chad passes by the foot of the bed.

"Dada." He must be at Helena's door. "I called for Mama."

"Mama's still in bed," Chad says and the words stretch

and groan. He must be picking her up. He must be hugging her. "So you get your ol' dad."

"Can I go in the big bed?"

No! She can't come in here. No snuggling right now!

I flip back the covers, slide out of bed, and run my feet across the floor like skating. I shut the bathroom door. I sit on the toilet and wait for my eyes to adjust to the glow of our nightlight. I open the drawer. Pull out test. Tear foil wrapper. Click test in holder. Pee. Pee. Pee more. Pee on hand. Recap stick. Tear off toilet paper. Wipe holder. Place test in drawer. Close drawer. Wash hands.

Mission accomplished.

I turn on the light and open the door and wash my face and put on my pajama bottoms.

Chad always says, "I just want it to be like it was the first time," whenever we talk about our difficulties in producing a second child. "It was magic."

He's right. It was magic. But it can be magic again even with the sticks, the pee, and all the Ninja skulks to the bathroom. It will seem like magic to him, and when it finally happens, it will feel like magic to me. It just. Needs. To happen.

Today might be the day.

I brush my teeth and put on a shirt. Two minutes down. Time to open the drawer.

Survey says!

O

Empty. No eyes and a smile. No happy face beaming, "You are good to go. I repeat, good to go!"

Not fertile.

No dice.

"Mama!" Helena says when she sees me come out of the bathroom. "I'm in your bed."

"I see that," I say.

I go downstairs.

Maybe tomorrow.

Tomorrow just might be the day.

2

i was twenty-eight and sitting with my knees against the center console of my 1967 Mustang. My back was pressing against the handle of the window roller-upper.

I was looking at Chad. He was tall and thin with boyish brown hair, and he drove an old Willy's and wore faded t-shirts with band names I had wished I had been cool enough to recognize. He also had a strong chin and an ability to keep his hands off other women's butts, so even though we had only been dating for about two months, I had a sneaking suspicion I had thwarted my grade-school predictions: I wouldn't be marrying anyone of Crotch-Pinching descent.

"So how do you feel about kids?"

Two months may have seemed a little early for the kids question, but things with Chad had been going so well; I had to know if this was going to be a snag.

"Having kids?" he asked.

Great. Stalling.

"Yes. The real deal," I said.

"There are a lot of ways to be involved in a kid's life," Chad said, "and I definitely want that kind of strong relationship with a child someday."

"Involved in a kid's life," I said. "You mean like Big Brothers and Big Sisters?" My knees slipped straight and one hand reached for the skinny steering wheel.

"Something like that. I just don't think you have to share blood to be a huge part of a kid's life."

I moved my other hand to the wheel and let my fingers dip in the lumpy underbelly of the hard black plastic. I ran my eyes along the shadows of the garage door.

"So... you don't want to have kids." I was too afraid to ask again, so I said it like a statement. A statement with a sag. A statement waiting to be corrected.

"Not of my own. There are enough kids who need good homes. I'll adopt if anything," Chad said and picked at something on the dash. "Why add to the population issue?"

Population issue? You've got to be kidding. Of course I knew there was a population issue or would be a population issue... someday. But that was filed in that far nether region of my brain in a guilt-encased Things I'm Supposed to Care About file—a file I felt good about having and fully intended to act upon once I was older and smarter and had more time. The slick of guilt around the file certainly wasn't enough to actually make me do something about it. Forego children, a desire that was orange and purple and searing, for the sake of an issue that felt as abstract as trying to peel an egg with soccer balls for hands? No way.

"That's assuming the kid you could have wouldn't be a part of the solution," I countered in my best unbiased voice. "I mean what if your child was the next Rachel Carson? The next Dr. King? The next Carl Sagan?" (As if any of these people could have cleaved their DNA from a mother with a Things I'm Supposed to Care About file.)

"Yeah. Maybe," he said flatly.

The conversation had looped outside of the personal. I didn't try to push it back in. But I did worry. Can it go like that? Can it be that a relationship is in so many ways perfect but can end over one thing?

"He'll change," an older friend and father of four girls told me. "We all say that. I said that. And look at me now." He gestured toward the four 11 X 14 portraits that hung above his sandstone mantel. "I'd never go back."

And maybe you don't do this, but sometimes or maybe all the time, without even knowing it, I hold onto what I want to hear. Even though I think I could kinda sorta maybe if I really strained, make out the faintest din of a crowd chanting, "Red flag! Red flag!" with the bi-colored and bare-chested passion of sports fans on crack, I instead listened to this one kind and dark-haired man standing with his arms akimbo. Yes, I had been told that one of the biggest contributors to divorce is people marrying under the hopes that their partner would change, but it didn't matter. I saw my friend's words slide from the slot under his nose like a receipt. I snatched it. And held it like a golden Wonka ticket.

He'll change.

Two years later, Chad and I started talking about marriage in the same forced way we had talked about kids. In the middle of an early version of this conversation Chad had been standing in the kitchen of our fifth-wheel trailer and had started opening cabinet doors without touching any of their contents. Lift, lower. Lift, lower.

"Baby," I had said, "why are you looking in the spice cabinet?"

"I'm looking in the spice cabinet?" Chad had said his eyebrows thick. He turned and we both looked at the jars tilted and wedged like sailors and whiff the b.o. of cumin spilled. "Just thought I'd, you know, make a quick stew."

We had laughed and it became our code name. Any time I wanted to talk about marriage, I would say, "Can we talk about the spice cabinet?" Because somehow that seemed so much better. Somehow one click away from the word itself, a makeshift synonym instead of the word marriage (which he seemed to really be picturing as MARRIAGE!!!) allowed us to strip the idea and cradle it in a new way. In a way that we defined.

By the end of a series of many Spice Cabinet conversations, whose penultimate had involved me giving what I grimace to call an ultimatum (I would never follow him to another town without a ring on my finger), he said, "Just don't bug me about it, and I'll do what I need to do to get there."

And that's where it began, I guess, a sense that certain things can be not talked about and even must not be talked about in order for them to come to be. And even though this was a new thing for our otherwise very open and leave-no-emotion-unanalyzed relationship, I trusted the silence. I never brought up marriage on its own or socked in a culinary euphemism. And by March I was wearing an engagement ring.

That following summer we had a routine. We'd leave our trailer, cross the tracks that glowed east-west in the setting sun, walk the tidy grid of numbered and lettered streets of the college town, and somewhere by his favorite breakfast joint I'd say, "Let's check mail." And Chad would roll his eyes and say, "Do we have to?" and go along anyway.

One evening Chad had just hit up the ATM, and I said, "Let's check mail," while he was still stuffing his bills in his wallet and maybe wouldn't notice my forearm on his guiding him to the right.

"But we never get any mail," he said.

"But still."

"Oo, Pennysaver, here we come!" he said with his neck extended and his hands fanning out next to his ears. Chad has brown eyes and the same expressions I'm sure he had when he was six and digging dirt tracks for his trucks or twelve and planning where to hang a rocket in his room. Even though I hadn't known him then, there are times when he makes gestures like this one with its sarcastic enthusiasm, when I feel like I had.

We were already halfway down the block, the post office door in sight.

"You never know," I said and smiled.

"Really? For real, what is it about the mail?"

"Honestly?" I said. Chad may have unexpectedly walked by our open bathroom door once just as I was removing a tampon such that he asked me, "Why are you holding it like a dead mouse?", but this whole mail thing was even more embarrassing.

"Seriously." Chad stopped.

My hand was on the metal of the door and Chad's other self was tall and dark in the glass. I let go of the handle and looked at Chad's eyes and the way his hair always sailed two antennae toward the back of his part like they were picking up alien frequencies. Working on his engineering thesis all day? Try sending transmissions to the Mother Ship.

"The thing is…"

"What is the thing?" Chad smiled.

"The thing is… something big is going to happen," I said.

"In the mail?"

"Maybe in the mail. It's just that I'm always waiting, knowing something big is about to happen." I looked at him. "Something great."

It's not that this was a new thing. I had had it all my life, a feeling that I would be sooled out, maybe get that note in class that told me to meet with the principal who had decided I was the most _____ student in school and that he needed my help. Sometimes as an adult I'd round the bend of a hallway and expect to see this person there waiting to give me orders to go _____. It didn't really matter what the thing was as long as it was something happening, that I was being picked out of the hoards and recognized as being The One.

I laughed. Chad laughed. Then he put his arm around me and got quiet and stood with his eyes like Wyoming kidhood afternoons scanning alleys for fort-building wood. "Perhaps you are about to receive a mission," he said. His eyes were serious now, squirrels turned wolves tracking rabbits from behind trees. "It's a letter that reads, Dear Tracy, We are looking for people with extreme sleuthing skills and a love for whales; you were recommended to us. Should you choose to accept this mission, you will be given a map and a partner—"

"A dog."

"Yes! A sleuthing dog trained in the art of map reading and cetacean study. You will meet him on the corner of Third and B tomorrow 11:36 a.m.

"However, if you accept, you must not tell anyone about your mission." Chad's mouth closed; his lips went inward; it was a mouth waiting to breathe again.

"Not anyone," he continued. "Not even your fiancé." His eyes swiveled to the side. To me.

Being selected for a mystery that involved whales and a secret dog partnership? Talk about an easy choice. "Sorry, Baby."

Chad laughed. "Then are you ready?" He pinched the brass PO box key between two fingers.

I took it and opened the door. I took it and loved him more. I took it and felt so lucky for finding someone who would come inside my silly dreams and breathe them into life. I held the key and knew I could tell him anything even if it meant I would not be telling him about my secret missions, my dreams-come-true. And in that shiny linoleum-floored world inside the post office, my choice—my dream over disclosure—only felt like it brought us closer. We valued each other's dreams so much, we would cheer each other on at the cost of silence. And like the Spice Cabinet decision, this silence and the trust it demanded felt like part of our foundation.

"Pennysaver," I said as I pulled out the flimsy magazine.

"But you just never know," Chad said and swung his arm around me.

"You never know," I said and leaned into his chest and tossed the Pennysaver into the green bin.

When Chad and I got married, I stopped using birth control. Without arguments, or tears, or discussions about overpopulation, we had agreed to have a child. I'm not sure when Chad had changed, but he had changed, just like my warm-eyed friend had anticipated years ago. And maybe this should have surprised me, but really his change only confirmed the story of how I knew my life was supposed to go. I am meant to have two kids. Of course he had changed.

After six months without using birth control I was still not pregnant. It seemed a little weird. I had gone online and learned about these over-the-counter urine tests you could do called ovulation predictors. I asked Chad what he thought. "Too forced," he said. "I just want it to happen naturally. On its own."

"But it doesn't seem to be happening on its own," I said.

"I'm not saying don't use them," he said. "I'm just saying I don't want to know about it."

I, too, thought the "happen naturally" paradigm was ideal. It should just happen on its own. But I was also starting to freak out. I was thirty-three and getting ever closer to that thirty-five-year-old cutoff when, according to doctors, statistics would go against me. My last gynecologist had held a ballpoint between his blond-haired fingers and had hashed two arced lines on the crunchy paper of the exam table. "Here is the risk of you having a child with genetic disorders. Here is the risk of an adverse affect to an amniocentesis. Where these cross," he had said and stuck the tip of his pen on the center of the bowed X, "is at age thirty-five." Thirty-five—dong! I could practically hear the echo. My gyno had gone Long Duk Dong on me and seemed all too satisfied to bear the news. And apparently his point was this: a pregnancy before thirty-five is like a whistle-filled skip down a *Bambi* tableau (minus the rifle), full of flowers and fuzzy animals, and nimble creatures with tidy hooves. But at thirty-five pregnancy becomes like a Jason movie full of creaks and clangs and slow pans on pitchforks, and decisions about who's going to check out that noise in the shed.

Of course I was going to use ovulation predictors. Thirty bucks and some pee every morning? Screw natural. I just won't tell Chad I'm using them if he doesn't want to know.

In my first cycle of using the sticks we had happened to have sex the night before the test looked positive, so the day of the positive I didn't insist on another round. I was going out of town and I didn't want to make one of those frantic calls to Chad's work and have to meet him at the door in some ransacked slut gear in the hopes it would smooth things along. (That would come later.)

When I had not gotten my period after two weeks, I bought a digital pregnancy test on the way to the gym. I walked through the locker room, which was full of old women pulling on swimsuits, laughing and leaning and reaching for each other's arms. The bathroom stall at the end of the row was empty. I peeled open the box and peed on the stick and rattled the toilet paper dispenser to make it seem like I was doing something in there. Something other than waiting.

"Pineapples, margarita mix," said a voice. A stall door creaked. A shoe appeared. It was one of those through-and-through tan jobs as smooth as a horehound with the sugar sucked off. "You know, just the cheap stuff," she was saying. Ol' Horehound was listing the ingredients of a cake, and any second now she'd say condensed milk; condensed milk had quite a fan base in the aqua-aerobics crowd. "One box of green jello, and"—she paused; her heel lifted and foot pivoted (come on, don't let me down!)—"a can of condensed milk. Not evaporated! Condensed."

Yes!

Pregnant.

Yes!

What?

I looked a second and third time. Pregnant. Pregnant. I bought a second test on the way home.

Pregnant.

Even though I couldn't feel anything, no outward bumps or inward kicks, I was different. New haircut kind of different. Or first-day-of-school different when I'd push my new-socked feet into my brand new shoes. Different. And maybe a little shiny.

That evening I picked Chad up from work and suggested we go out to eat. I was driving and he was telling a story about work and I handed him the stick whose screen still had my new word on it.

"What does this mean?" he said, smiling.

At dinner he'd wad pizza to both cheeks and through a flap mouth like an advent calendar say, "I can't believe it."

"I know," I'd say.

But I could believe it because, why not? I was pregnant just like a million other women. Pregnant like I knew I always would be. At eight weeks we told our families, and it wasn't until Chad's sister told him that we may want to wait until thirteen weeks before telling anyone else that I even considered something going wrong. And even then I was just annoyed she had rained on our parade when the meow-meow was already out of the sack.

After the first ultrasound, Chad and I named the baby Lima Bean since we didn't want to know the gender. We also didn't want to know if there were any genetic disorders.

"We get what we get," Chad had said, and here was that nature theme again. But I agreed this time wholeheartedly and felt fullness in our ability to promise love, real love, to a legume silhouette.

Lima became Helena when she was born. I had laughed after I gave a final push and heard her screaming, laughed at the relief, a strong, healthy baby. Laughed at the joy.

Chad had gotten teary-eyed and looked at her like she was a new planet or a species just discovered at the edge of the world.

At the time I didn't wonder what that might mean, those two separate and very different reactions. But later I would remember them, later when Chad would talk about Helena's birth. "It was the most amazing thing I have ever been through," Chad would say and still says when he talks of her coming into the world.

Obviously Chad had really changed from the day of our driveway talk years ago. Not only had he been willing to have a child, he had been awestruck by the experience. And as much as I was glad for this passion (Helena would have a devoted father, and I would be able to call on this passion yet again when it was time to have number two) there was something I hadn't anticipated in this joy of his coming around. It is something that I hear in his voice that I don't have in mine, some ounce of the miraculous that I lack.

Pretty hard to feel miracles with your knees around your ears and your rectum turning inside out, I try to justify. But I still feel guilty, as if for laughing upon her arrival, it means I love my daughter less. Then I feel challenged as if Chad and I are on opposite sides of Helena, looking at her with nothing but beauty, and looking at each other with something to protect.

It's like another friend told me when I was pregnant.

"You may love your spouse more than anyone in the world, but you will love your children more." And as much as I think this isn't true exactly, that's only because I can list reasons it's not. In the visceral sense, in the way of a body plain aching, it's absolutely true. We all know who'd be the first hoisted on a chunk of flotsam if we were bobbing in Titanic's footprint. It's just how parenting goes.

So do I miss the simplicity of the other love, the all-the-time-in-the-world, sparkly-eyed, only-for-you love, when I would be the person nobly slapped on the chunk of floating wood in the biting sea? Yes. Would I undo my dethroning? Never. And does any of this mean I don't want another child? Not at all.

3

"You seduced me," Chad says as we lie in bed.

"Really?" It wasn't like I hadn't been trying to seduce him, but it surprises me, hearing him say it, hearing how easily it came to him like my actions had seemed plain, light, spontaneous even. Does he really not know?

"Oh, yeah. That was not what I had planned for my evening." Chad folds his arms behind his head and stretches them flat to the pillow. He smiles.

Am I being dishonest? Do I tell him my motivation? Do I tell him that even though this morning's test was an empty O, I know that any minute now my luteinizing hormone will kick into overdrive and the follicle maturation race will begin? Do I tell him that surely by tomorrow morning the grey circle on my ovulation predictor will be filled with two eyes and a smile, which means that even as we speak an egg is probably getting ready to fling itself into the warm embrace of the fringy fallopian tubes? Do I tell him that I know it's coming because earlier in the day I had wiped and seen a slick of clear mucus?

He is still grinning, looking at the ceiling. His eyes are closing.

Can we do something about the word mucus?

"Guess you just never know," I say. I raise my eyebrows. I smile. And I am in another life; the words have time-machined me back, and I'm in a life we used to have. We will lie in the dim coziness of our intimacy. Maybe he'll get up for water but will come back to bed naked and we'll talk or watch a movie or just lie here remembering and forecasting secret things, together things. One of us will say something like, if you could have anything to eat right now, served up right now, what would it be? And he'll say buttered popcorn and I'll say, with real butter, or from-the-pump movie butter? And he'll say movie butter and I'll gag, and say, no way! And we'll laugh, and he'll say how about you? And I'll say funnel cake. And he'll say strawberries or no? And it will go on like this in its silly importance. It will matter. It will matter more than anything.

But this matters, too. This matters more. An egg could be flinging! Sperm are right now swimming! There are things to be done and tended to. I don't want to mess this up!

"Can you go let the cats in?" I ask.

"Why?" Chad whines and rolls over and shoves his face in the pillow.

It's a cruel request, especially since if it were up to him, he would leave them out. But I want them in. I want them in and there ain't no way I'm gonna risk this precious payload dropping out of the Ironman going on inside my vagina. Just keep swimming! Find the golden egg!

"Please?" I ask and bend my knees to maximize pelvis tilt. That's right little spermies, let gravity be your guide! If I sling my feet to the ceiling, will it be too obvious?

Chad flips back the covers and pulls on pants. He is still smiling and his hair is messy and his skin is so smooth and without the freckles I have. He is quick to tan in the summertime, was one of those boys who'd shave his head when school got out and in August even the buzz was blond and his skin was dark from so much sun. I would have loved him then just as much. Would have seen him in some candy store with one of those banging screen doors and he'd have been standing in front of the Skittles and Reese's Pieces trying to decide with his fingers pinching his lower lip or pulling on his chin. I would have tried to say hi.

"Thank you," I say.

There he is. Here he is. Standing with his pants and no shirt. Standing like he was when I finally did see him for the first time. Not in a candy store but a gas station. He had been wiping his hands on a rag. Stay. Stay here. Stay in this place where the thank you just means thank you for letting the cats in, and thank you for the great orgasm and thank you for asking if I wanted my funnel cake with or without strawberries.

But this thank you is a different kind. This thank you is heavy and really an apology for what it is I cannot be.

It's a thank you for what he does not know or is pretending not to know, but a thank you for playing along anyway, a thank you for riding this bus.

The next morning I slide out of bed and run my feet across the floor like skating. I shut the bathroom door. I sit on the toilet and wait for my eyes to adjust to the glow of our nightlight. I open the drawer. Pull out test. Tear foil wrapper. Click test into holder. Pee. Pee. Pee more. Pee on hand. Recap stick. Tear off toilet paper. Wipe holder. Place test in drawer. Close drawer. Wash hands.

Mission accomplished.

I turn on the light and open the door and wash my face and put on my pajama bottoms.

Today might really be the day. After last night, a perfectly pulled-off seduction enjoyed by both parties? It should be the day.

I brush my teeth and put on a shirt. Two minutes down. Time to open the drawer.

Survey says!

O

No spike in hormones, no flinging egg, no smiley face affirming that everything works and that, yes, I'm fertile and I've done everything right.

I eject the test in the trash and shove it down the side so it cannot be seen. I wad toilet paper and shove it on top.

Chad appears at the door messy-headed and squinty-eyed with nothing but his briefs on.

"Too bright," he says and turns off the light and in the darkness steps behind me. He wraps his arms around my shoulders and stays squeezing with his chest pressed to my back. "That was fun last night," he says. And even though I cannot see his face, I know he is smiling a hooked smile pulled to one side.

I dip my legs so his arms drop. "I've got to go make breakfast."

I go downstairs.

4

When I had gone to my gynecologist a year after Helena was born, I said, "I stopped breastfeeding three months ago and I still haven't gotten my period."

She said, "You're probably pregnant."

My doctor was a salt-and-pepper haired woman who would bug her eyes so you could see 360 of white around the iris when she listened and alternately drop her lids flat when she talked. The effect was that you felt like she was soaking in your every word, but actually your syndromes and concerns were no big deal. "But, Doc, I keep feeling this pain…" (eye-bug, eye-bug). Eye-drop. "Normal," she'd say, her lips spreading flat. This would happen often enough that I started wondering if Dr. Flapp thought of me like this woman Chad and I used to call Crutch back in Davis. She had been a short-haired elderly woman who'd hobble the streets with one crutch and seven appendage wraps she'd rotate across her body. Wednesday? Broken neck and meniscus blown. Thursday? Brain tumor and bunionectomy, Friday? Just your run-of-the-mill disembowelment.

But maybe if Flapp thinks I'm usually a hypochondriac but now thinks I'm pregnant, it means I really am. Pregnant already? Wow. Cool.

"Let's take a look," Dr. Flapp said like she was flipping channels or about to give her Stouffer's a poke.

She pushed around my abdomen and got the urine results from the lab. "Nope, not pregnant," she said and scrawled something on a pad. "Here's a prescription for birth control. It's pretty hard to have a newborn while you have an infant."

I took the slip and drove to the CVS nearby and fingered the As Seen on TV merchandise while the prescription was getting filled. I thanked the woman as I reached for the crinkly white bag. I drove home and placed the bag in the bathroom next to a set of second-string towels, but it wasn't until I saw the bag tilted there all eager-to-please that I felt a little sorry for it. I'm not taking the pills. I had never planned on taking the pills. I'm all for being logical and planny-planny and let me put it on my Outlook calendar, etcetera, but go on birth control and risk having it stay in my system somehow? Hell no.

Six months later, when I still wasn't pregnant, I was out of the if-it-happens-it-happens stage and into the any-day-now-would-be-perfect stage. The age-gap issue seemed increasingly important to Chad. He didn't have a lot to say about the actual second kid, but when I'd bring up a sibling for Helena, he'd say, "Anything more than three years apart seems a little far. Definitely a four-year gap is the max."

It was time to step up the game. I bought an ovulation predictor kit, but in wanting to save money, I bought the kind where you have to compare two blue lines. I didn't realize you had to be an art major or a forensics expert to read the damn things.

The second line should be darker in color. Not thicker, not fuzzier. Just a more intense hue. It should be clear.

"Chad," I said one morning, desperate for a second opinion and knowing he could keep it clinical and not get into a big discussion about the use of tests. It wasn't my using the tests he was opposed to, but knowing about them, having discussions about them, or having the sense that they dictated our sex life seemed to be the turnoffs. Test drama raised resistance. I tried to keep my question light. "So what would you say about those lines? I don't want to sway you, so you look and tell me how you would compare them."

He took the stick. He squinted. He held it up to the light. "One is blue. The other is blue, but a little bit wider."

"Intensity. We're supposed to be looking for intensity here."

"This one is more intense, but it depends on how you define it because–"

"These things suck," I said. I snatched the test out of Chad's hand. I had been peeing on the sticks for three weeks with the expectation that this would be my certainty, our certainty, that would get us what we want. I couldn't deal with any haziness in the very tool that was to bring us our sure thing.

"Yeah, fuck them," Chad said. "Fuck Clearblue Easy."

"This isn't funny," I said. "It's supposed to be easy. Just tell me when we need to do it and we can do it! What are we supposed to go dropping thirty bucks a month just to find out when we kinda sorta maybe might be ovulating? It's pretty bogus."

Some weeks thereafter we were at a party and I met a woman who had two kids who seemed pretty far apart in age. I had to ask. "So how old is your daughter?" This was always my starter question, the question I would use to feel them out. Maybe she had planned to have them far apart or maybe she had been through the very thing I was experiencing.

"My daughter's four and my son is three months."

Within minutes I was spilling my guts.

"We haven't used birth control for a year-and-a-half and I'm just wondering why it's not happening." I tried not to look desperate, but I could feel my face going comic strip: mouth like an upside down kidney bean, frantic circles ringing my eyes.

The woman told me about a book. She called it her fertility bible. She threw a few words at me like mucus and egg white and luteal phase. I had no idea what she was talking about. This was good. Something to know.

I got the book and read it in three hours, read it in a green chair pushed up to our dining room window. And it wasn't that the book was biased, but in explaining the details, the careful dance of hormones that make the ovum mature inside the follicle and burst through the wall, the feathery come-hither gesture of the fallopian tubes that guide the egg inside, I starting wondering how anyone gets pregnant. So many factors have to be aligned and happily in sync that the odds of getting pregnant seemed worse than winning the Lotto or landing a dime on a cake plate at the fair.

But I could do this. I would do this! I took note of all the signs of ovulation: the clear stretchy mucus, the softening cervix (the book even had a picture, and I hate to say it, but remember the ends of those cheese-filled hot dogs?), and the shift in temperature after ovulation had occurred. I made copies of the empty charts in the back of the book and filled in a row of dates. I was ready. I would keep track of my body, take daily logs, become so aware that I would actually start feeling (as my mom claimed she could feel) the minute one of those little eggs started busting down the chute.

I circled my temperature on the chart each morning. I field-noted the consistency of my mucus in tiny penciled writing. I X'd the days we had intercourse. And unlike just peeing on a stick and waiting, the daily charting gave me something to do and gave me the sense that every day was worthy of data collection. I was like an astronaut in training. Beam me up! And presto-change-o one day my temperature did shift. It works! My body is doing exactly what the book described!

But the careful monitoring of my cycles revealed some things: they were long, typically between thirty-five and forty-five days, and one month there wasn't much of a temperature shift. After three cycles I was still not pregnant. I went back to Dr. Flapp.

"What day are you?"

"Twenty-eight."

"So you definitely should have ovulated."

I had read about this in my book as well, the assumption that every person has a twenty-eight day cycle.

"Actually, I have long cycles," I said while Dr. Flapp's eyes bugged. Yes! She was listening. I pulled out my charts, three sheets of paper whose lines and circles looked like the football plays my brother used to draw on the back of napkins. "Maybe you want to look at these? I've been charting, so I know I'm ovulating, but maybe not every month. And my cycles are long."

Her eyes dropped. "Most women ovulate around day fourteen, so we can give you a blood test to make sure. But you should probably take Clomid. How old are you?" She glanced at my chart.

"Thirty-six."

"Most women your age have a hard time. With the Clomid we can know exactly when you ovulate."

Had she just not heard me? I don't ovulate on day fucking fourteen. And what's with Clomid? Why would I take it unless something is wrong? And if something is wrong, shouldn't we actually try to diagnose and fix it before just throwing drugs at a giant question mark? Granted, I may be biased since my mom's cure-all was hot lemonade in a Peter the Rabbit mug. Sore throat? Menstrual cramps? Poison oak? Ingrown toenail? Flat tire? Try hot lemonade! But even with Mom's narrow pharmaceutical scope in mind, Dr. Flapp's quick reach for Clomid without even looking at my diligent charting data seemed flippant and even irresponsible.

"I'd like the blood test."

"Let's do the blood test. And make another appointment when you're ready to talk about Clomid."

When the nurse called with the test results and I had ovulated, Chad asked, "So what do you want to do?"

I noted the "you" in his question and had the sense he would do anything, that he was along for the ride. And as much as I wished he would have a greater take, that he would actually help me with the decision, I was relieved he was not saying no to the Clomid. Or worst case scenario, saying no to the bigger thing that felt like it was swaying over our heads like a fat piñata stuffed with family portraits that did not yet exist: Helena with a new baby's feet pressed to her cheeks, me with a baby in one arm, Helena in the other, all of us at the beach walking and making a perfect line of four.

"I just feel weird about the Clomid. Why was that the only thing Dr. Flapp had to offer?" I said and dropped my eyes and held an imaginary chart. "Call me when you want to talk about Clomid." I mocked Dr. Flapp's southern accent and made it extra thick.

Chad just shook his head.

"And why would something suddenly be wrong with me? We can get pregnant. We have Helena."

"You're fine," Chad said. "We're fine."

And with that I wanted to go the other way, say, maybe we're not fine, though.

But it seemed like a reaction borne of the same stuff I used to feel as a teenager when my mom, based on hours of me drawing in my room, would later be telling someone, "And Tracy loves to draw," after which I'd pipe in, "Not really, Mom. Not anymore." I'm not sure what that was, a desire to be mysterious? To never be summed up? Or maybe Chad saying, "You're fine" just fell into one of those no-fly zones. It felt similar to me saying, "I don't even really want this cookie," as it was on its way to my mouth and him saying, "Well, maybe you shouldn't eat it then." There are some seemingly innocuous things with their tagalong implications that just shouldn't be said. And as much as I appreciated Chad's confidence or maybe his attempt to console, what did it mean? Did he not want me to do the Clomid? What if I change my mind and want to throw myself on Flapp's prescription pad next week?

"I think I want to stick to the charting. Maybe have another conversation in six months if nothing has happened," I told Chad and looked away.

But it will happen. Of course it will happen. How can it just not happen?

Chad put his arm around me. Pulled me so my shoulder fit under his armpit perfectly. This is good, right? Hugs, arms slung over the shoulder, quiet looks across the room? This is good silence. The same kind of silence as the Spice Cabinet; the kind of silence in which things happen, good things. I felt the weight of his arm and stared at the kitchen wall.

I'm not sure if it was later that night, or in one of the many similar nights that followed, but sometimes as my fertile days approached I'd grow anxious and fearful and full of doubt. And silence wouldn't be enough. We'd be lying in bed and I'd want to call a huddle with Chad, devise our strategy as a team: "Okay, I may be fertile any day now," I could picture myself saying, bent over a clipboard and drawing a bed with naked limbs sticking out in odd contortions, "so we need to start hitting the sheets." But he doesn't want to know the details, I'd think. He doesn't want to know the plan.

But I want to talk to him about it.

If you tell him you'll ruin the mood.

But why should I be the only one who is worrying about this stuff? Why does he get to be left in the dark?

Because sdhjkasf;kajsdbti.

What?

He doesn't want anothewekhwihefbfurwu.

Forget that. What's the goal? What do you want from him?

Seed. I want the seed.

Then don't say anything.

And even though I could feel that keeping my trap shut would be the right thing to do, and even though we'd be lying in bed, lights out with Chad's breathing shifting to the long sluggish breath of sleep, momentum would build in my throat with the weight of a thousand moons.

"Do you even want another kid?"

Chad's breath would snag, "What?"

"Do you want another kid?" I'd say.

"We've talked about this," he'd say and stretch.

Buying time. Stretching is never really stretching in

these kinds of talks. "It has been a while," I'd say.

"What was it, four months ago?"

"It just seems like you don't even want another kid."

"I do want another kid."

"But there's that thing in your voice."

"There isn't a thing. I've already told you."

"What?" I'd ask.

"I'd be happy if it was just you, me and Helena, too."

"So you don't want another kid." I'd say and could feel my head bob on each word.

"It's not that I don't want one. It's that I'm okay if we don't have one."

"But that's like saying you don't want one. Like some spirit up there in the universe is really going to want to come down to our family if you are indifferent."

"If the spirit is going to come down, it is going to come down. It will choose us. It's not like we aren't trying," he'd say and roll over.

"We could be trying harder." I'd feel it in my throat and I'd want to stop. I'd feel my vision getting narrower, me sinking into a hole darker than our room. I'm wrong here. I know I'm wrong. "We only tried, what, four times during the last window?"

"That's the best we could do. That was the best I could do," he'd say, and I would already want to apologize.

There are things we have been so smart about, things we know in a marriage are smart to do: still saying please and thank you, still kissing goodnight, agreeing not to go to lunch alone with opposite-gendered coworkers unless we were already friends. For as much as these things seem trivial, and as much as our bond feels unconquerable, we have seen the way love unravels if you do not tend to it, choose it, hold it in the palm of your hand like a small bird.

But we have done this. We have introduced this thing, these other people: one frenzied and driven and the other indifferent and pressured, and we have asked them to make love. When they can't make love, we ask them to have sex. When they can't have sex, we ask them to fuck. When they can't fuck, we ask them to copulate. And in the end we, or I, just want them to breed. Is this dangerous? Are there ramifications to pimping ourselves out in the name of a goal?

"I'm proud of us. We're trying here. We're doing what we can," he'd say and I could hear the defensiveness in his voice. I should have apologized. I still can.

"I know," I'd say in the quiet trail off way that meant I was done talking. And again I would wish I were different; I would wish I could say, "You're right, good job" and really mean it.

These conversations still happen, and I still feel like I have in the past: as long as there is one opportunity lost, I know that if I get my period I will feel like we have failed. I will know we could have done something more. I'm aware of the irony: in deadening the act to mechanics, we are trying to create life. But there are facts here: the egg is alive for twenty-four hours and sperm can live up to five days. It's a pretty damn small window. And I can't feel good about our process if we don't get the right result. I can't feel good about anything until I am that big-bellied woman all feet splayed, waddling down the street with number two on the way.

As dumb as it sounds, I keep thinking about that opening scene in *Top Gun* when the shaken-up pilot drops his wings on the desk. I know the tightness he's talking about; I can feel it in my chest like fists of insistence that only one outcome is possible. And even though I know how tightness and holding on can flip back on itself and lead to the opposite of intentions, what does letting go mean? Accepting that this may not happen? That we may not have a second child? That Helena will forever be by herself out on that log?

No way. I can't let go.

5

i slide out of bed and run my feet across the floor like skating. I shut the bathroom door. I sit on the toilet and wait for my eyes to adjust to the glow of our nightlight. I open the drawer. Pull out test. Tear foil wrapper. Click test into holder. Pee. Pee. Pee more. Pee on hand. Recap stick. Tear off toilet paper. Wipe holder. Place test in drawer. Close drawer. Wash hands.

Mission accomplished.

I turn on the light and open the door and wash my face and put on my pajama bottoms.

Today might be the day.

I brush my teeth and put on a shirt. Two minutes down. Time to open the drawer.

Survey says!

O

I eject the stick in the trashcan. I look at it: dumb white plastic, a yellow peed-on flap like a tongue. I tear two squares of toilet paper from the roll and place each one on top of the test like a shroud. It's a shroud waiting to burn on a pyre of trash. Burn, pyre, burn.

I smile.

I am okay. Today, for some who-knows-what reason, the slim thud of dread does not come. The weight of grey, of not knowing, of not passing tests, of uncertain futures, the bile of disappointment does not crawl into my lap and curl up.

I turn and see Chad standing in front of our closet pulling out a shirt. He looks at me.

"S'up?" I say and tip my head.

"S'up Dawg," Chad says and hits his chest and moves his hand like a palsied bird.

In a parallel universe Chad and I are rappers.

In a parallel universe, I am infertile and okay.

I walk to Helena's room. "Where's my Little One?" I say as I pull open the gate. I toggle her bedroom lights to an orange glow. She moves her head and I can hear her hair scratch her pillow; it's long and wild hair that knots like a nest at the base of her neck.

"Too bright, Mama," she says and pulls the covers over her head. I pull back the covers and climb in next to her.

"It's time, kiddo," I say finding her ear with my lips. "It's time."

"Noooo."

"Yes," I say and kiss her ear. "Okay, deal with your dad. I'm going to make you guys Creamo."

When Chad and Helena come downstairs, Helena says, "Creamo!"

"With lumps," I say as I put the bowl in front of her. "But it's hot."

"Stay in the shallows, Dada," Helena says to Chad like she's forty-three and he's six. "It's hot."

"Good batch of Creamo," Chad says looking over his spoon.

"The mix-ins," I say and smile. "It's all about the mix-ins."

I take a sip of coffee. Maybe it's good if I don't get pregnant this month. We still have a house to move into. Maybe it would be good to just take a break from it all. It will happen soon enough.

I give Chad and Helena hugs as they get ready to leave. I stand behind the glass door and watch as they walk to the car. Helena climbs in and Chad stays standing next to her open door. His mouth is moving. He smiles and straightens. He cocks his head, brings his hand to his chin, pushes his lips out and cinches his brows to make one thick line. The dude's a walking Muppet. He snaps to with his finger wagging and all serious like he's just solved an equation, but a corner of his mouth is starting to curl. Hard to stay in character when your little girl is cracking up. He shuts the door. As they drive away, Helena turns her head to see me. She holds up a finger and bends it like a worm taking a bow. I do mine the same.

This feels good.

Maybe tomorrow I won't even pee on a test.

I go upstairs, open my computer, and sign into my email. I have a message from Sarah.

The title of the message is News.

News.

Shit.

When I was seven, or maybe eight, I was friends with a girl who had a shiny brown bob and doe eyes. She wore dresses and tights and ribbons and socks with lace on the edges and her name was Maria Gaziano. Maria lived in a white house that had one of those wood plaques dangling from the front porch awning that said "The Gazianos" and we walked there often after school. I don't remember thinking Maria rich the way I sensed rich when I was a kid—moms who were home after school and made Tollhouse cookies or served little bags of chips with cans of Coke and had laundry running that smelled like Bounce. But Maria did have something I did not, some order to her life that showed itself in the row of Victorian dolls that sat on a high shelf in her room, hair and dresses as if they had never been touched, and in the lace bundles of candied almonds Maria had gotten from all the weddings in which she had been the flower girl. I didn't envy everything about Maria, but I did want that thing, that tidiness, that certainty, although back then I didn't know that's what it was. Instead, the thing I saw was her girliness. I wanted that. The dresses and the shiny shoes, the poster on her wall of a toe-shoed foot with shiny pink ribbons x'ing themselves up the ankle. Maria took ballet and had a tutu. I wanted that.

"I want a tutu," I told my mom, who was only beginning to come out of her hippie faze even though she still wove macramé plant holders, listened to Joni Mitchell, and loved every shade of rust. "I like earth tones," she'd say in her defense.

I couldn't blame her. In marrying my dad, she had been a military wife during the real hippie era, and when my dad and she had divorced, she had to make up for lost time. She'd never go to a sit-in or bang signs around the Berkeley campus. She'd never ride a bus up the coast, get stoned with a bunch of intellectuals and throw pots on a commune. A kerchief tied on her long brown hair, wearing a lot of jeans and flannels, and attending a few Save Sandy the Whale! meetings may have been as close as she would ever get.

"But you don't take ballet," Mom said and I could sense the waver at the end, that she hoped, but kind of knew this wouldn't be enough.

"I know. Maria says there are classes at the rec center." This was sketchy territory; Mom wouldn't know what to do. She was not a fan of anything girly even though I can't remember anything explicit she ever said or did that made me so sure. Maybe it was the way she dressed me in my brother's brown and green hand-me-down Toughskins and on picture day would agree to tying thick pieces of primary-colored yarn, never ribbon, around my ponytails. Or maybe it was just the way every kid knows about his or her parents, through that kid osmosis—all those unlogged hours of watching the side of a parent's face while they drive, or listening to the way their voice changes when they talk to the grocery checkout person, or seeing the way their mouth goes thin when you ask if Brenda Hatcher can spend the night. It's those million pieces of data about what they value and what they do not taken so consistently and unknowingly that by the time you are three you know who your mom is talking to when she picks up the phone.

"I think people start ballet when they are three," Mom said.

"But Maria takes it."

"When did she start?"

"I don't know."

"Are you saying you want to take ballet?" Mom asked.

Of course I want to take ballet! But don't make me say it! But I had to say it; if I didn't she would not take the hint. And also I knew, even as I felt myself getting smaller and felt a lump in my throat that was thick with some kind of betrayal, that Mom loved me. If I said I wanted to take ballet she would have to let me or otherwise let her own bias stand plain.

"I guess so."

"We can look into it."

"You don't want me to take it?" I could ask that now. She had already said yes.

"It's not that!" Mom said with the push of two brows. "My mother made me take that stuff, ballet, cotillion. I hated it. I don't know why she always wanted me to do that stuff. And then she'd curl my hair."

"Can I get a tutu?"

"Let's see how you like it first."

I don't know how much I badgered her or if I had to badger her at all, but she did sign me up for lessons, and she did buy me a leotard. It was a peach Danskin long sleeve. Unfortunately I couldn't talk her into the peach tights or even white tights. So I sat in the passenger seat of my mom's Chevy Chevette and pulled my Danskin over the only tights I had: bright red cable-knit jobs that looked like a sweater for legs. I was doomed. Also, my mom had warned me that it was a beginning class and the other students were probably a lot younger than I was. "That's okay," I had said. (I'd probably just be better than everyone else. More skill with age.)

So I walked into the room with mirrors and yellow sun slanting through the large arched windows, and while I'm sure my mom said goodbye, in memory I only feel her drifting away as I stared at the ring of girls sitting and stretching on the wood floor like tiny petals flung on the ground. They were small. I was big. Each had her hair pulled back in a tight ponytail or bun. I had fluffy curls dangling around my face. And they were all so pink. And I was… I was… peach and ketchup, and even worse, knit ketchup with little pills balling up along the thighs.

The teacher introduced me and had us stand in a circle. "I want you to crouch in a ball like a tiny seed. Picture yourself being a seed all dark and warm under the earth." She had us do it then. I closed my eyes and was relieved to no longer be standing where it was so obvious that I was a tractor in the orchids. "I will tap one person on the back and that person will sprout and dance around the circle, blooming into a beautiful flower, and she will tap the next seed on the back and so on. Are you ready?"

I was so fucked. Of course I didn't know it then. I was actually trying to think of how I would grow, what I could do to blow them all away. I didn't know any fancy moves, couldn't pull a triple Salchow or double Lutz, but I would dance, I would let my arms come out and I would be the prettiest flower of the bunch.

The music fell, heavy piano then oozing strings. Maybe the teacher would pick me first. I opened my eyes enough to see one set of pink slippers gone. Someone had already been picked. If I focused on the music, I could turn into something, I could be different somehow and they would see it. I peeked again. Two pairs of slippers left. Now one. My tights pulled at the knees so my skin looked like tiny squares through the thready hatch of red lines that felt rough on my cheeks. It had to be my turn soon. I closed my eyes. I had to be good. I was last. They'd all see. I waited, squeezing my arms around my shins. I waited. I opened my eyes. The slippers were gone. All of them. Slip-shush, slip-shush, big feet were hurrying toward me. One black slipper cut the lines of wood. The teacher tapped my back.

I did something. I must have done something, some halfhearted saunter around the ring of tiny girls whose heads were turned and watching and me wishing in a million ways I were any place but there.

"I want to quit," I said when I slumped in the maroon vinyl of the passenger seat.

"Are you sure?" Mom said.

I never went to another lesson.

But in the story of life, it's not about the ballet lessons that never happened; it's about what happened in the instant I saw the black shoes, about what became clear.

The girls do not want to tap your back. You are not one of them. They do not want to see you dance. The teacher probably doesn't want to either, but she has to. All of those things I heard without realizing I was the voice behind them, such that they rang out like a million truths. I don't know if I can blame genetics or being the second born or that I had dropped my entire Burger King chocolate shake on the pavement when I was riding home on my bike, but it's as if my interpretation of events even at such a young age had to go that way. Already I was headed for the pity pot, and even though I had and would continue to have an irrational hope of something really big about to happen, and even though I would later have enough good things happen to really believe the right thing does evolve, my first go-to would always be of the lone rider getting screwed.

I had seen this before in myself, seen how the extremity of giant hopes and the abyss of pity left me living life like a coin two-sided and pitched in the air and always waiting to land. It was anyone's guess, certainly not my own, how it would come down. I thought I had started to change that about myself, started to round myself out, hope less, do more, fail more and tell myself that was okay, too.

But Sarah's e-mail. With the e-mail I am seven again, standing on the outside in my red tights, wondering why me.

I don't want to open it.

Sarah is a member of the five-woman mom's group I had been in before we had moved. It was a group, formed not by lifelong friends, but by the group's central member, Tina, who had picked us off from various encounters since we each had a child around the same age as hers. The ten of us would get together once-a-week so the kids could play and bite each other's toys while we talked about pulling up and crawling and walking and whether or not to try Potty Training Boot Camp. In this way, the group was perfect. These women were kind and smart and grounded, the kind of women you could call if you needed babysitting because you had a doctor's appointment or because you were about to launch your kid across the room if you didn't get a second of space.

That's what people always offered anyway, and although I felt comfortable cashing in on the offer when I had to go to the doctor, and while I felt comfortable confessing sanity loss after rationality was regained and the heat of madness had long since cooled, I never felt right calling while in the thick of it. It's not that I feared judgment or backstabbing, but I guess I feared the emptiness, the lack of the right expression. I didn't want a loose hug or a hand on the arm or a head tilted with an "I know what you mean" patching it up. I wanted the woman who would get in the trenches with me, ask me the tough questions, follow and push me on my conjectures and theories, laugh with her mouth splayed open and get me to laugh at myself. I wanted the woman who would cuss and cry with me.

I wanted Tracy. Tracy with her red hair and trapeze smile and the smack-sucked quietude of her mouth on the end of her highlighter as she edited all eighteen handwritten drafts of the paper that was due in six weeks. We had been roommates in college and after college. We had also rowed together, kissed the same boys, popped each other's zits and nearly clocked each other's lights out and still came out friends. And as different as we are as people (I'd still be typing the only draft of my paper ten minutes before class), in some ways our shared name fits: Being around Tracy has always been as easy as being with myself. Most of the time easier.

I didn't have this kind of thing with this group of women. And as much as I knew that friends like Tracy are rare finds and that it takes time to build meaningful relationships, I longed for something more personal. However, at least it was nothing like the first mom's group I had been in; that group had been nothing but awkward. I'd be sitting on the floor all kumbaya style with four other moms and our babies undulating in front of us like those battery-operated animals they used to pen up in front of Spencer's Gifts at the mall. We'd be sitting in silence, gaping silence, and I'd start hoping someone would choke on a nut or at least vomit on Grandmother's hand-dyed quilt just so there'd be something to say. When one of the women started throwing out comparisons about the kid who hadn't been able to make the group ("You know, it's funny, Jackson is older than Theo, but Jackson can't roll over yet!"), I decided to bail.

Maybe it's hard to get to know women within in the context of motherhood, I started thinking, since motherhood is cloaked in responsibility and good choice-making and an effort to always be one's best self. Where's the intimacy in that?

But then one afternoon while we were sitting in Tina's bright living room, Lynn said, "Is anyone else going to start trying again?"

Finally! I thought, knowing exactly what she was talking about. Someone's getting to the goods!

Four of the five of us wanted another child. Sarah told us she had already had one miscarriage months ago. Lynn was going to start trying. And although Tina also wanted a second child, she wanted to wait until she felt ready. She also wanted to time it so the second baby would be born around the same month as the first so that if she had another girl (which she hoped she would) she would already have all the properly fitting seasonal hand-me-downs. The two-month-sized snowsuit would fit. And so would the three-month-sized Valentine's dress with the appliquéd hearts.

This bugged the shit out of me. Who does this kind of planning other than my grandparents, who spaced their children in four-year intervals to avoid tandem college tuition? And who sticks to the plan even as months roll by and Sarah gets pregnant and miscarries for the second time, Lynn finally gets pregnant and miscarries, and month after month I have nothing to say but, "Nope. Still trying"? Who actually has this kind of choreographed thing come true? And who can afford to disregard fear?

Stand by for a reality check, I thought, when Tina finally announced that their kickoff would be January, that she and her husband were going to start trying this month. "I hope it works for them," I told Chad later that evening as we stood in the kitchen doing dishes, "but shit just doesn't work that way."

"Maybe it will," Chad said.

"Maybe," I said. "But after everything we've been through and Sarah and Lynn have been through? I just can't imagine even thinking that way." I shook my head.

One afternoon when it was just Tina and I at the park, she asked, "Have you thought about other options?"

"My gyno says Clomid. I'm too scared of multiples," I said. I didn't want to go into the other reasons, all the cosmic reasons Clomid just didn't feel right. The fact that we'd be stressing ourselves on a timetable and risking the one-in-ten chance of multiples for only a thirty percent success rate. The fact that were we to get multiples, we'd be faced with the decision of how many to keep. The fact that we might feel more reckless somehow if we used a drug to force the release of an egg that could result in a child with extreme health issues. Health issues are always a concern, but would we feel more responsible about a child with health issues who was the result of my incentivized eggs? Or about the two kids who were a result of the process when we only wanted one? If the outcome were anything other than the one healthy child we wanted, would we have regret? And even bigger, since we already know we can have children, would using Clomid somehow feel like playing God, like we were trying to manipulate our fate? It's not like I had it all figured out; I certainly didn't know where the actual life of the child, where the soul came from, but I wanted to believe that it was some kind of partnership. I wanted to believe that Chad and I would provide the love and the body, and a soul would choose us and let us be its host this time on earth. I liked the complicity of that idea; it didn't feel so unilateral. And I liked the idea of being chosen and granted an opportunity by something larger than a drug that makes my body think it's low on estrogen.

When she asked again a few weeks later, "So is the risk of multiples your only issue with the Clomid?", I wondered if my approach to getting pregnant was bugging her as much as hers was bugging me. Was she wondering where my logic was? Wondering why I didn't have a backup plan?

"I think I'll give it till summer," I told her. "Then maybe consider the Clomid." But I didn't really mean this. Well, I meant it in that part-truth way, as a thing to say that seems normal and sane. But really I was giving myself a fat inner wink-wink the whole time. I wouldn't use Clomid by summer. I wouldn't have to. I'd be pregnant by summer. I just knew.

"Have you thought about adoption?" Tina asked and held her daughter's sippy cup with both hands.

"Not really." I had the impression that adoption was a lengthy and expensive process, but mostly I hadn't given it much thought. "The thing is," I looked at Tina and felt my shoulders pitch forward, "we can get pregnant. We know everything works. We have Helena."

I turned and watched Helena chasing Tina's daughter around the slide. Helena is beautiful. Beautiful and healthy and funny and kind with hands that point to things and small fingers that rest on my arm. And she just came to us without doubt or fear or stress. She happened; on her own she happened. Why would anything have changed?

Tina didn't say anything, just flattened her mouth and looked at her own daughter.

We were not good enough friends to question each other's approaches, or maybe my lack of logic didn't, in fact, bother her. Or maybe she was fighting her own annoyance because, like me, she had realized that the path to pregnancy is too personal, too spiritual, for anyone outside of the couple involved to toss in any two cents.

But this is the danger in sharing. Although in talking to someone about infertility, there is a wonderful release, a sense of not being alone, the cost of not being alone means there may be comparison. In this case, I have heard and said myself, "I'm so glad she's finally pregnant, especially after everything she's been through," as if one person's miscarriages warrant her more happiness than the person who had no difficulty. I have a friend who spoke of her sister saying, "I mean she expects sympathy because she's struggling to have her fourth child! I can't even have one!"

And while I know the feelings are normal, and while I have them all the time myself, I am tempered by the reality of my own desire. I already have one child. I should feel complete just to have her. But I don't. I want the chance to hold a baby again who is my own and do it for the second time when I am less afraid. I want to see how that baby is different and feel what it is like to share such intense love for two distinct beings. I want to know it's possible to love that way twice. And I want Helena to have a brother or a sister. The ache is real.

So do we disregard the pain of some and validate the pain of others? Do we try and quantify pain through numbers: number of children already had, number of years of trying, number of miscarriages, how far along the miscarriage was? Do we try to dissect and delineate and categorize simply because that is how the brain works or because we are trying to bring ourselves comfort through trying to fit the world and ourselves on a graph? In the end are we just trying to defend our own pain?

"I just want someone I know to get pregnant and to have a normal pregnancy," I said to the group one morning. Sarah smiled and nodded. "All these issues we are having. It just seems weird." It was weird. Three out of five seemingly random people not able to get pregnant or see a pregnancy through after already having one child without any issues? It seemed like a lot.

I really did mean it when I said I wanted someone to get pregnant and have a normal experience, but of course I hoped it would be me. It wasn't just because it's what I flat out wanted for myself, but in some remote way I also liked the idea of being the first in the group. I wanted the kid but also the heroism of turning the tide of misfortune. I wanted to be the breaker of the bad luck so I could ride in front of the masses all blue-faced and kilted and lead everyone to their big-bellied peace.

In March, I found out that's exactly what would happen. Move over Mel, here comes Mama Love.

I had bought the test on the way to Jack's third birthday

party and had kept it in my purse the whole time we stood at the park under a grey sky, sung happy birthday and cut a cake that looked like Thomas the Train. Helena was exhausted when we got home, so I gave her milk and we read two books and she finally fell asleep. I rushed to the bathroom, peed on the test and set it on the window sill.

If it's negative I can always try again with morning pee. If it's negative, that's okay. I unfolded and refolded towels on the rack. I looked in the mirror. It really is okay. I smiled at myself. I leaned in, so many gray hairs. When did all these happen? Mom didn't start going grey so soon did she? If you're not pregnant, you will just keep trying. Don't worry. Women get pregnant at forty-two. You'll just keep doing what you're doing. I looked at the digital display.

Pregnant.

Pregnant?

Pregnant.

I'm pregnant!

I walked into the bedroom. Chad was sitting in the bed with covers around his waist. His shirt was off. He was going to take a nap.

I edged in next to him and handed him the stick.

He took it. Looked. Paused. "What does this mean?" he asked, his mouth tight.

It was the same thing he had said when I was pregnant with Helena. They were the same words, exactly the same, yet entirely different.

"I guess it means I'm pregnant." You idiot! I wanted to yell. A trap door thumped open in my chest. What's his problem? Doesn't he want this? Shouldn't he be excited?

He handed the stick back and lowered himself under the tide of blankets. "I'm just scared."

Scared of what? Scared of a miscarriage? Scared of your own disappointment? Scared of mine? But there was something else he was scared of. I could see it in the way his head didn't turn. See it in the stillness of his hands.

Chad rolled over.

I looked at his shoulder cut to a triangle by the brown sheet. I left the room.

By the end of the week I called the doctor to make my first OB appointment. The woman on the phone said congratulations, the kind of congratulations you give someone after they have completed something, a congratulations without strings or doubts or things left unconsidered but instead like a fat red mark checking an empty box. "We'll see you in six weeks," she said.

"Should I call if there is any spotting or anything?"

"A little spotting is probably normal, but anything more than that, call."

But there wasn't any bleeding. Just more nausea. And I started sleeping in jog bras because my nipples felt so sore.

"My boobs hurt," I said to Chad one night as I was putting on pajamas.

"You sound pregnant."

"I am pregnant."

"I know."

We still hadn't talked about it. Just let him go through whatever he needs to go through, I kept telling myself.

Just like the Spice Cabinet. Give him time. But I had started feeling the dark stone of resentment. Can't we start talking about room rearranging? Can't we turn out the lights and lie with our heads together on a pillow and whisper about names?

"When are you going to tell people?" he asked.

"After the doctor's appointment. What do you think?"

"I don't want to think about it until after the doctor's appointment."

"Why do we have to act like it's not happening?" I said. "It's good news. Can you and I at least acknowledge it instead of being so negative?"

"I'm sorry. I'm just not ready to believe it until after the doctor's appointment. When you come home from that and everything's fine, I'll be on board. I promise."

"That's fair." I had filled Chad's ear with stories of the women I knew and all the difficulties they were having. I could understand why he would want to stay guarded. Maybe he was just afraid of loss.

But I was pregnant for crying out loud! I could feel it. Beyond the classic signs, I could feel a little spirit walking with me in everything I did. I stuck to my spin class and when I would start getting tired, I'd feel a surge of energy as if my new friend was saying, "Not so fast, there, Mom, don't give up now!" and I'd smile at the burgeoning tenacity unfurling in my womb. "This kid's a little scrapper," I'd think and pedal faster.

One evening when I was in the kitchen chopping an onion, Helena held up a puzzle.

"Want to do puzzle, Mama?" she asked. Her eyes are

brown like Chad's.

"I can't, kiddo, I have to cook. Excuse me." She didn't move, just stood and looked at the box in her hands. I stepped around her. She walked down the hall.

Moments later I heard the thump and skid of her coming. She passed through the kitchen with her hard plastic dog on a string and a little purse stuffed with books, markers, a pajama shirt, and she was wearing one of my Converse on her foot. "We're going to the park, okay, Doggie?" she said as she passed by.

I fail her. In so many ways, I'm not enough. I don't have enough time or enough interest to play like a sibling could. I can't make her laugh in that little kid way and be silly and goofy and jump on her bed making vowel sounds and put shoes on my head and paint on my arms and pour cups of water on the bathroom floor and say, "Look, I'm going pee-pee, sssssss!" and do it until the floor is slick and the steps of a big person are getting louder and louder and louder.

Four more days, kiddo. I'll go to the doctor and I will come home and tell you about the person inside of me. I'll tell you about the little person that will be yours, too.

The next afternoon Tina called and wanted to walk to the park. It was March and already felt like the coming of heat, a hazy blue sky with clouds pulled flat. Tina's daughter was on the green swing, swaying like a pendulum between us. Helena had run to the small yellow house.

"Helena really loves opening and closing that door," I said.

"I'm pregnant," Tina said and straightened her mouth

as if apologizing.

I am, too!

"That's awesome!" I said and gave her a hug.

"I just didn't mean for it to happen to me first," she said and put her palms up like a teacher had asked to see inside her hands.

Tina with her roll-out date. Tina with her plan. Tina with her wanting to wait so all the outfits fit. And it had happened. She had gotten pregnant in their second month of trying (which had been the same month as their first). And what we didn't know then, but would know eight months later, was that, yes, it would be a girl. Apparently shit could work that way.

Shit can just work that way.

"Just be glad it worked out for you guys," I said.

"I feel bad," she said. And I could tell by her wide eyes and sloped shoulders, she really did. "I just didn't mean to be the first in the group. After everything you guys have been through, it should be one of you."

"People in the group are just going to be happy it's going well for someone. I think at this point we all just want to see someone having a normal experience. I'm happy for you guys," I said, and was relieved there was no choke behind it, no grab of pain or jealousy.

Don't think you're so enlightened, there, Buddha. You're just not jealous because you're pregnant, too.

But I'd be happy even if I weren't pregnant.

Your better self would be happy, but you'd still feel a sting.

I wanted to tell Tina my news. I wanted to relieve her

of her heavy eyebrows and wrinkled smile, and I wanted to celebrate, to share, to swap due dates and thoughts on how to tell our daughters. I wanted to giggle and be dumb.

Three more days. In three days you will go to the doctor and then tell Tina, and you will both look back and laugh at this moment and how badly you wanted to tell.

"Well let's take a look!" Dr. Flapp said and let her eyeballs stay buggy as she shut my file and left her hand on top.

I undressed and lay on the table. The room was dark save the yellow line of light under the door and the small screen lighting our faces like we were in a movie or at a sleepover clustered around a four inch TV. I'm not sure what the joke was, but there was some sort of joke Dr. Flapp was telling. She was moving the wand of the ultrasound so the lit wedge on the screen looked speckled and blotched. Where was the fetus?

"And I'd see these military wives who had to wait until their husbands came off of deployment," she was saying and the nurse was listening and there was some punch line, a stunted sentence with space left for anticipated laughter at the end. I didn't know what she had said, was too busy trying to decipher the fuzz on the screen, but I could feel her look at me, so I did some kind of huh-huh half laugh and felt her face turn.

"Uh-oh."

But the nurse was still kind of chuckling and the room still hummed with the ghost of a joke, so maybe I had missed the punch line and the "uh-oh" was part of the joke. Maybe we were actually meant to laugh now, after the uh-oh.

I looked at the doctor, the lines on her forehead and eyebrows so dark. The room went so quiet. Why did the room go so quiet?

"There's a problem," Dr. Flapp continued, her voice was without a lilt or her usual southern drawl. "There's no heartbeat. This is the pregnancy," she said and pointed at a circle on the screen.

What? Wait. Keep talking. I looked at a dark sac on the screen. When you talk something exists. When you talk something has words. Keep talking.

"There's no heartbeat, and it just doesn't look right."

That's okay; just tell me more. What else do you see? What else can you do?

Someone knocked and cracked the door. "Sit up," the doctor said and covered my legs. She went to the door and the person on the other side whispered something about labor, delivery, need you right now.

"I have to go," Dr. Flapp said and flipped on the lights and took off her gloves.

Wait, it's done? We're done? That's it?

"I'm so sorry," she said. Her hand was cold on my arm. "But I have to go. I will give you a call this evening to talk about where we go from here."

I looked at the nurse. "You can get dressed now," she said and handed me a box of Kleenex. "I'm sorry." She left the room.

I stayed still. And sat. And let my legs flatten in the cool slick of lubricant.

The paper crinkled when I finally stood up.

Chad said he could tell when he saw my face through the glass of the front door.

Helena could tell, too.

"Are you sad, Mama?" she asked as she stepped onto the porch.

I knelt down. I wrapped my arms around her and squeezed her perfect little body with its warm and beating and strong little heart. You have a heart that beats and moves blood around your body. You have a real, beating heart.

I put my mouth next to her ear and could feel the cool edge of it on my lip. I'm so sorry, kiddo. I'm sorry.

Chad and I lay in bed that night. I rolled on my side. He hugged my back.

In the morning he got up and I said, "Do you mind if I call my mom?"

"No, please do. I'll take Helena to breakfast." He stood in the doorway. He scratched at the paint on the doorjamb with his finger eyelevel. "I'm sorry."

"I'm sorry, too." But I wasn't sure what we were sorry about, if we were sorry about the same things. It didn't really matter.

"Hello?" Mom's voice was quiet and soft. She was in another time zone, so she'd still be under covers. Her room would still be dark. She'd be able to hear seagulls if she listened or the sea lions on the foggy pier.

"Mom," I said. It was the same way I had said it when I was thirteen and caught for shoplifting, seventeen and dumped, twenty-five and thinking that if I just didn't wake up one morning that would be okay. Mom. Always Mom.

Tracy cried, too, when I told her. And both times despite my sadness I felt so lucky to have people, these strong women, to climb inside my pain.

I didn't say anything to Tina. Not right away. But I told Sarah and I told Lynn.

I had joined the miscarriage club.

Months later as Tina started showing, Lynn said, as we all sat on the floor, "I'm pregnant." She smiled with her mouth closed and rolled her eyes to the side as if trying to restrain her absolute joy. But she couldn't. She was stoked. And even though I did feel a pinch of pain, I told myself this is good. Momentum is shifting the other way. The tide is turning. Two out of four pregnant. Only Sarah and I left.

In September Chad, Helena and I had moved, and I couldn't go to playgroups anymore. But I was still receiving group emails and it made me feel a part of things even with the distance.

But this "News" email from Sarah? News can only mean one thing.

I open the mail and skim until I find it.

Pregnant.

I back up and read the sentence: "Hanging out with Tina and Lynn must have rubbed off on me because I'm (finally) pregnant again."

Oh.

I look away from the computer.

I read the mail again. It's a group email addressed to all four of us. There is the sentence, "Hanging out with Tina and Lynn must have rubbed off on me…".

But I can't hang out with Tina and Lynn! I want to yell. I can't bask in the oozy-oozy pregnancy pheromones that are dense and fissioning and swarming the neighborhood such that even spayed cats are wide-hipped and slinking to their prenatal yoga class with their mats across their backs and their soy decaf teas warming their paws while they purr at having their fertility back! I am missing out on the pheromone cloud!

And I'm not pregnant.

I had never even considered the danger before: What happens if you form a sense of a group around an identity no one wants to be? What happens if that identity changes for some but not everyone? What happens if I am the only one left forever? If I never do get pregnant?

Then just be you not getting pregnant.

Don't think of yourself as "the only one" or "the last one." Don't be the girl in the ring of ballerinas who didn't get picked.

"Yippee!!!" I type after I hit reply. "Could there be any better news?!!!"

6

My mom always said I could do anything. I can't remember a specific event, an inspiring squinty-eyed time when she said it and I got back in the ring, but she said it, must have said it a lot, because it stuck with me. You can do anything you want to do. There wasn't a lot of talk about what that anything might be; I never felt pushed or driven into a specific career. But there were certain tracks set forth by tacit expectations. College was a given. Mom used "when" in talking about college, not "if." And there were always those kids she'd brag about, some other person's kids who were "biking across Europe" or "backpacking in Nepal."

She'd say, "You know Steve at work? His daughter is—"

"Let me guess, biking across Europe?" I'd say and roll my eyes.

She'd laugh and say, "Yeah, can you believe it? Italy, actually. Doesn't that sound fun?"

It did sound fun, sort of. But I couldn't really tell. Every time I'd think of it, try to picture waking up to the sun beading the seam of a Tuscan hill, I'd hear Mom's bluebird enthusiasm, "It's a beautiful morning! Tweet, tweet! It's a beautiful day! Isn't this exciting? Today you're biking across Italy!" such that I couldn't really picture how I felt about it on my own.

And about marriage? Mom said, "Your dad and I were too young. Make sure you can support yourself first."

So explicitly or not so explicitly my takeaway was this: get an education, wait to get married, have a career, and bike across Europe. Or maybe ride llamas across Turkey. Or go live in a yurt.

I'm not sure how you'd do the research, but I'm guessing a lot of girls growing up in the eighties got a similar thing—all the fallout from women who had or had not taken advantage of the choices they had finally been given. Women who had maybe just missed the cusp of choice or who only at that time knew of a few girls who didn't get married their senior year of college, become secretaries then housewives. "It's just what we did," Mom would say. And then she'd get wistful over a girl in high school who had read *Time Magazine* and was in all honors classes. "Why couldn't I have been more like her?" Mom would ask. And as a kid I'd feel weird about her longing for a different choice, ultimately a path that would undo my brother and me, unzip our DNA and launch our existence back into the cosmos.

"But we wouldn't be here," I'd say to her.

"Well that would be awful," she'd say in her mom voice.

"You guys are my biggest accomplishment. My biggest life's work."

And I'd feel glad to have her back again and be glad to have returned to the center of her world.

But as I got older the same conversation would go a little differently. I stopped saying, "But then we wouldn't be here," and she'd stay in the regret of her adolescent self and keep the camera rolling. She'd bump through college with familiar scenes: dark-haired Danny, Johnny who said he loved her but didn't, reading Camus under an autumn tree, taking walks in the rain. I could never see her memories very clearly, even though I had heard them enough, but they were hazy and clichéd as if testament to her claim: "I just didn't even know who I was then." And if we kept talking I'd hear about the marriage, the divorce, the staying in California, the return to school, and this is where the momentum would build. Something would shift in Mom, her mouth would go thin and her voice academic, confident, and in catching up to present day and reflecting, she'd have a summary: "I mean I certainly see my life about more than just being a mom. It's not the only thing that has defined it."

I could see how she meant it. My brother and I were both her biggest accomplishment yet not everything her life had been about. If I stayed on the literal level it made sense. But if I tried to reconcile the emotion behind both (on one hand sheer awe and gratitude and the other a kind of reined-in resentment) I felt confused. Mom didn't really know how she felt about motherhood? Or maybe she just felt all of it.

So given these contradictions, maybe I shouldn't have been surprised on that balmy evening when she was visiting, but I was. I was thirty-one years old. I had gone to college. I had taken a backpack to Europe by myself, and even though I had come home early, we all blamed it on the rain instead of on my loneliness. I had taught three years of public school, become a Divemaster, lived alone, travelled to Honduras, Mexico and Belize. I had maintained my relationship with Chad while volunteer teaching for a year in Ecuador. When I returned, I moved in with him and found a teaching job and started looking into grad school. Mom had driven up for the weekend.

"Your eggs are dying."

"What?"

We had been talking about my relationship with Chad, how long we had been together, how I knew he is whom I wanted to marry. She had asked if we had a timeline and I told her yes without the details. We had pulled up to the curb and gotten out of the car. The sky was losing its color. The sun was pushing long shadows from the trees and the buildings, from the triangle of mom's nose. And she had said this thing about eggs.

"What are you talking about?" I asked.

"You're going to have a mongoloid."

Her face was stunned, too, eyes big, mouth small, like she had just burped an awful thing, a thing that had obviously zipped right by the ol' grey matter.

"Did you just say mongoloid?"

"No. You know what I mean."

"Not really."

"Your eggs. They get old. If you wait too long, they start dying. You won't have any good ones left." Mom was talking fast, her eyes still wide and both hands clinging to the strap of her purse where it crossed her chest. Her elbows were in, her body stiff. And she, the women's studies teacher who actually used words like "people of color" and "marginalization," had just said "mongoloid." Clearly, this was serious shit.

"I can't believe you said mongoloid."

"I meant— "

"Down's Syndrome?"

"I know. It's awful. It's what they used to call them."

We walked into the auditorium to watch one of my students in a dress rehearsal of *Swan Lake*. We found seats and the lights dimmed and we did not speak. But as much as I had tried to redirect the conversation, what buzzed between us was not her political incorrectness; it was dying eggs. Were they dying all the time? Were they dying right now? How many would kick the bucket during this one shabby performance of *Swan Lake*? I was scared. And then mad.

Even though I had done it all, felt like I was doing it all: education, career, independence, travel, it suddenly didn't matter. I was thirty-one, and apparently the whole time I had been hiking Cotopaxi and diving with hammerheads in the Galapagos, little headstones had been popping up all over my ovaries and turning them into rocks. Obituaries were being penned about the hundreds of half-souls who had never even had the chance to live! What happened to "Have a career"? What happened to

"Wait to get married"? What happened to "Bike across fucking Europe"? Because at the end of the day, this is what it comes down to? This is the bottom line? "Oh, P.S. Be sure to squeeze kids in there somewhere because if you don't you'll have a mongoloid."

As I go through this struggle to get pregnant, I am not alone. I am surrounded by a surprising number of cohort women: women in their thirties who are educated and have careers, women who have traveled, had broken hearts and broken the hearts of others, women who have found or not found the right person and who finally want to have kids. And what is happening? They can't get pregnant. Or they get pregnant and have a miscarriage, or two, or like one good friend, three. I'm not sure what to make of this. Are we all the product of a shortsighted group of feminists who stressed the career over the family? Are we the victims of poorly planned sex education that stressed the dangers of getting pregnant and not the risks of an infertile future? Are we the product of a society that gives us so much choice that we want to do it all? Are we the product of our own life's success that, until now, has told us to set goals and they all will be attained?

But I did everything right! I did everything I was supposed to do! And I feel like I'm standing on top of a mountain yelling into the wind.

I'm not sure who to be mad at, but I want to be mad at someone. Because if I can do anything, why can't I do this? Why can't I get pregnant?

We got through the rest of Mom's visit without talking

about eggs, but as soon as her car was out of the driveway I ran to the computer. Maybe I could find something on the internet.

Three hours and two cups of coffee later, I was white-faced and slack-jawed.

"I think we need to talk about the Spice Cabinet," I had told Chad at dinner, my mouth still feeling like one of those dummies that sits on a skinny guy's leg and doesn't have the lips to articulate words. But I didn't tell Chad why. Poco a poco, I thought. Little by little.

Looking back, I know Mom's visit was the first time my assumptions were rocked. It was the first time I actually thought of my body as aging and having the potential to thwart what was otherwise meant to be. But it was only a lifting of the veil; it was awareness racing around my impermeable bubble of truth. It was enough to cause me a cerebral fear, the way I might keep off chicken for a week after reading a headline about someone dying of Salmonella. But I didn't actually believe it. Like so many other fears, it stayed chatty in my head while in that quiet and hidden place in my heart where all the dark things live, Morse Code was tapping out in the flutters between beats: not you, not you, it will never happen to you.

7

i slide out of bed and run my feet across the floor like skating. I shut the bathroom door. I sit on the toilet and wait for my eyes to adjust to the glow of our nightlight. I open the drawer. Pull out test. Tear foil wrapper. Click test into holder. Pee. Pee. Pee more. Pee on hand. Recap stick. Tear off toilet paper. Wipe holder. Place test in drawer. Close drawer. Wash hands.

Mission accomplished.

I turn on the light and open the door and wash my face and put on my pajama bottoms.

Today might be the day.

I brush my teeth and put on a shirt. Two minutes down. Time to open the drawer.

Survey says!

O

I eject the stick and shove my hands in the trash. I grab tissues, Q-tips, a tube of mascara, yesterday's peed-on test, and I shove. I shove with straight elbows, pushing until the bag slips off the edges of the can and starts to wilt around my forearms. I shove until there's no more room, nothing gives and everything that can be made smaller is. I stand. I wash my hands. I rip off one long strip of toilet paper and wad it up and drop it in the can. It's like a flower. A lovely trashy bloom.

I walk by Helena's room. Chad is kneeling by her dresser talking to her about whales.

"Mama, are whales your favorite?" Helena asks.

I go downstairs.

After Chad and Helena leave and I am cleaning up the dishes, I get a phone call. It is my stepmom.

"Yes, you guys should drive up!" I tell her.

There is a delay on the cell phone, or she is just pausing, then she says, "I'll talk to your father. I'll let you know."

My dad and stepmom have this dog. She's a fine dog. She's a pretty dog. And according to them, she is the smartest dog on the planet. Well, according to them, she isn't actually a dog. In fact, if they were reading this they would wonder what dog I was talking about.

They have never left the dog in their lives. Yes, they will let her stay home and watch television if they go to a movie, but if she's in the car, my dad will stay lounging with her in the back seat stroking her head while we all go in and get burgers.

The dog is now sick. And while I am worried about them (especially for my dad whose sentences keep ending with "I just don't know" and the silence of a long ellipsis)

I am secretly excited that her sickness has meant boarding her at a specialty vet six hours away. They have to leave her there for the weekend. Darn.

"We'd love to have you see our new place," I tell my stepmom. One of the perks they hyped when Chad found a job in South Carolina instead of California was that we'd be closer to them. We could now be a day's drive away. And with both of them retired, it was easy to picture weekend trips or rendezvous at the beach. But the dog kept feeling like a complication. Not only does she have an unpredictable past with small children (a.k.a. nipping the air when they run by), she has a nascent interest in chasing cats, and I didn't know how to explain to ours that the Rhodesian Ridgeback once used to hunt lions in Africa was only visiting. But no dog? No problem. "I mean we still don't have a lot of furniture or anything, but it'd be fun to see you guys."

When my stepmom calls back, she says, "We set the Garmin for your house. We're on our way."

"Great," I say. "See you soon!" I hang up.

Oh shit—it hits me then—they'll be arriving in the Fertile Zone.

My seduction two nights ago was successful but pointless, so I must be extra vigilant now. I saw a four inch string of precious egg white mucus fall into the toilet this morning. The ovulation predictor's face was empty, which means I know it will smile soon.

But it's not like my dad and stepmom are going to know anyway, right? It shouldn't matter that they'll be here. And with our new extra stout queen-sized captain's bed being delivered today, they won't even hear the headboard. Maybe it will even make things more fun, in that let's-pretend-we're-in-high-school-with-our-parents-in-the-next-room sort of way. Or maybe it will fill Chad and me with a sense of teamwork: us versus the unsuspecting AARP members! At the very least it will feel like a secret.

"Guess you'll have to give that new bed a stress test!" my dad says and elbows me in the side and laughs. They've been here for three hours, and we're sitting at the kitchen table waiting for Chad to come home from work. Ha, ha. Ha,ha,ha! I laugh, too. I laugh extra hard so my face will glow red and cover what would otherwise be an obvious blush. My god, does he smell the pheromones? Does he sense my desperation? Does he know that every morning I've been staring at that dingy gray screen praying to see eyes and a smile?

Just four months ago I was visiting them and spilled the beans about our efforts and the miscarriage. I stayed general and put together, trying to be careful about not saying too much.

I fold a napkin and try to recover. My cheeks start to cool. He doesn't know anything. He's joking.

"Yes, don't worry," my step-mom says, while her blue eyes spread large and her hands move like they are smoothing an invisible table cloth. She keeps speaking but slowly, like she is building a word mosaic or explaining how to catch a bus to a tourist with a heavy limp. "We do not mind at all if you have sex any time while we are here."

Is this really happening?

"I was already saying to your dad—"

There's more?

"on the way up here: What if we are arriving during their fertile time?"

Holy shit.

Do you remember that scene in *Sixteen Candles*? When Molly Ringwald's character is felt up by her grandmother? I am her face, all eyes and a little o for a mouth. And what am I supposed to say? "Thanks for the green light! I'm actually going to be fertile any minute now! Anyone for a bet? Wanna double down if we do it doggy?"

This is not good. I nod. Try to chuckle. If only I were the kind of person who could think fast during these situations, maybe say something like, "Great, we'll get fucking!"

That's something Chad would come up with. "You don't lie, exactly," he's told me in the past. "You just take what they say and validate it or exaggerate it." But, not ol' Trace. I'd like to think it's the curse of being too damn honest, but right now it just feels like a curse.

I say something, mumble something about "purse… jacket…. shoes" and try to cut myself off before I list every form of outerwear; "rain gear" sails past my uvula heading north. I stand up and leave the room. And as I look into the gaping darkness of the hall closet and feel my cheeks pulsing such a convincing lighthouse impersonation that I can actually hear a foghorn and taste salt and smell heaps of dying kelp, I decide I need to get something upstairs. Surely there's a scarf or hat or mitten to attend to.

Chad has always been careful about who he tells things to. He says, "Once you've told someone something, you have no control over what they do with the information." I think of him now. Thank god he wasn't home to hear what just happened in the kitchen. No doubt he'd raise his eyebrows and look at me as if to say, "See what I mean?" I can hear kind intentions behind my stepmom's public service announcement, but telling someone you're worried about crashing their fertile week? Probably not a good idea unless you know you aren't crashing their fertile week.

Chad finally comes home, and we go to dinner and get Helena to bed late. We stay up talking and I practically tuck my dad and stepmom in since I'm glad to have someone staying in our extra room. It's a nice change, having other people, other humans to talk to. It's a nice break, getting out of my head.

When I get in bed, my body hurts with fatigue. I close my eyes.

"Look at us," Chad says. "Look at us in this snazzy bed." His voice is too loud for being on the brink of sleep.

"Pretty crazy," I mumble.

"I mean we're really stepping up in the world."

We have never actually owned a bed frame in the eight years we have been together. "I know," I say.

"And nightstands!"

I can't respond. This kind of dialogue could very well end up with us rolling around in the hay in that let's-celebrate-how-far-we've-come way. And that's exactly what I want, right? Every night I've been trying to come up with some new way to make sex seem organic to our evening just so a good bank of sperm will be thrumming north by the time the ovulation predictor pings smiley in the morning. But for four mornings now there has been no smile.

Which is why tomorrow will probably be it!

But I'm... too... tired.

"This always happens," Chad says. "I am always wide awake when you are tired." (Translation: "I always want to have sex when you don't.")

My eyes are too heavy. What are you doing? He's ready to go! This can be it, the one time you have sex all month that will make you pregnant! How will you feel two weeks from now when you get your period?

"Sorry," I tell him. Everything goes black.

I slide out of bed and run my feet across the floor like skating. I shut the bathroom door. I sit on the toilet and wait for my eyes to adjust to the glow of our nightlight. I open the drawer. Pull out test. Tear foil wrapper. Click test into holder. Pee. Pee. Pee more. Pee on hand. Recap stick. Tear off toilet paper. Wipe holder. Place test in drawer. Close drawer. Wash hands.

Mission accomplished.

I turn on the light and open the door and wash my face and put on my pajama bottoms.

I brush my teeth and put on a shirt. Two minutes down. Time to open the drawer.

Survey says!

Shit.

Shit, shit, shitty-shits! What the fuck? You've gotta be kidding!

But you couldn't do it last night, remember? You asked yourself and you were too tired.

Who cares! I should have anyway.

I do not eject the test. I leave it in its holder and set it in the drawer with the face looking up. I close the drawer. I open the drawer. I close the drawer. I open the drawer.

Two eyes and a smile.

Today I passed the test.

I go downstairs.

"How'd you like the new bed?" My dad says and laughs and reheats his coffee in the microwave.

"It was nice," Chad says.

Crap, it's already starting. My dad is going to foul this up. He won't mean to, but without knowing it, he'll take this bed thing too far and he'll crack some joke that will touch some nerve and thereby turn Chad off from the sex we must have today. My parents are taking Helena to the zoo, so it's the perfect chance. It's perfect and absolutely required. I just gotta keep cool. No big deal. It's just a chance to have the nooner of yester yore, a chance to relive the halcyon days in the trailer when afternoon delights were the norm. It'll just be an old-fashioned roll in the hay, nothing less and nothing more. Easy-peasy. Just keep your cool.

"Well I can kind of sense," my dad continues, his eyes squinting, his one hand pinching the air; he steps closer to Chad (my god, shoot me now) "that you all didn't give it the true test. The real go-to."

What's going on? Is everyone in cahoots? Does my dad know he just may have snipped the existence of his future grandchild?

Chad laughs. I walk away. I've got to stay out of this. Maybe I'm the only one who's stressed. If Chad sees that stress, he will know there is some other thing going on. He will feel the weight and pressure of my master plan. I have tried to hide it from him this time, have tried to give him the "magic" we had with Helena's birth, tried to create the illusion that everything is just happening naturally, casually, so that one day I can hear him telling someone, "And then our second came along," as if it was his or her spirit up in the cosmos who had finally chosen us without nary one bit of orchestration. But I have to get him in the sack!

"How late is too late to have her back?" my stepmom asks.

"Three, probably," I say.

"Mama, are you going with us?" Helena asks.

No, Mama is going to stay here and try to fuck Dada's brains out so you can have a brother or sister. "Nope! You get to go with Grandma and Grandpa all by yourself!" My cheeks hurt from the smile I've cranked to my ears. And in case my Jedi mind trick's a little rusty, I add, "You'll have to show them the lemurs!"

"Okay," my stepmom says. "That should give you some time to paint. Use the time to get some stuff done."

"Oh yeah," I say nodding. "We will!"

Even though we've billed this outing as a few hours of free babysitting so Chad and I can work on our house projects, I'm hoping that he has also taken all the talk of sanding and painting with a wink. With Helena gone and an empty house, maybe he, too, will remember those has-gone days of grad school. Maybe he will naturally be in the mood, or maybe we can return to the nostalgia that had started to bloom last night. I can hear a movie director calling, "Pick it up from 'Look at us in this snazzy bed'—action!"

I hug Helena and stay standing outside as my dad starts the car and pulls it out of the drive. I turn and can see through our glass front door an orange extension cord running up our stairs. An electric sander whines. Chad's working? He's taking this whole "opportunity to work" thing literally? What about us? What about a couple alone in their new house? What about the snazzy bed?

My dad taps on the horn as they pull away. I wave.

Just let it happen. Don't say anything.

But what if it doesn't happen?

It has to happen.

How can he just not know? How can he be sanding the stairs?

I step in and let the glass door hiss behind me. Chad is sitting at the top of the stairs bending to get the sander flush with the trim. He's got on black boots, safety glasses, red earmuffs, blue and white gloves—every form of protection a human can wear. Foreshadowing, anyone? Ain't no way I'm getting laid.

I close the front door.

He cuts the sander.

"Can you leave that open?" he asks.

He has no clue.

But you didn't want him to have a clue; that was the point.

But he should have a clue!

Just don't say anything. You can still make it happen without saying anything.

"No, I can't," I say and twist the deadbolt in the lock.

Just come up with something inviting, or do something cute.

"We have to fuck," I say.

Not cute.

Chad looks down. The sander is still in his hands. "Now?"

"Yes," I start up the stairs. He puts the sander down. I want to hit him. I want to hug him. I want to be on the same side. I don't want this weight. "I'm sorry." I walk by him and I feel sick. This isn't how it's supposed to feel. You can't try to bring life into the world when you're feeling like this. Why did you say it like that?

"Okay," Chad says. I hear him getting up. "I was just trying to use our time effectively."

"Hey!" I say and then stop myself. Effectively? What do you think I'm trying to do? You think trying to take advantage of the one twenty-four hour window we are given every thirty-five days to achieve the one thing we have been hoping for in the past three years is not using time effectively? Why have I been peeing on sticks every morning? Why have we been contributing to the Clearblue

Easy's bottom line every month if we are not going to even do it during the one time doing it is even worth something? But saying all this and risking a fight will only kill the odds. I take a breath. "Do you know what I am saying here? Why I am saying we have to?"

So much for magic.

"Yes," he says, and with the flatness in his eyes I know he really does know. But there isn't a way. We can't recover. "Come here," he says and sits on the bed. I don't want to. I'm still mad. But I sit. Chad rubs my arm. "It's not that all hope is lost. I just don't like that kind of pressure, that kind of presentation." And I'm wondering if he means my presentation, since my hair is in greasy chunks and I'm still wearing a pair of fleece snowflake pajamas. (Note to self: if you want to get pregnant, burn the fleece.)

"I know. I just don't know what to say. I'm trying to keep you in the dark, but it backfires. I get pissed off that I'm the only one who is doing all the stuff, testing, trying to make it happen. I hate the weight of it all."

"Why don't we transition?"

"I'll go take a shower."

We go through the motions. We try to make it fun. We try to avoid the awkwardness and rely on our foundation. But we are somewhere else. I can feel Chad's body, but his spirit is gone. Maybe it's in our past, maybe it's in fantasy, maybe it's in some other woman who doesn't wear snowflake pajamas, but it's not here and it doesn't matter. It doesn't matter.

One thing matters.

"Thank you," I tell him. It's the same kind of thank

you and apology I said three nights before. Thank you for being strong. For not getting mad. For not thinking I'm crazy. Thank you for riding this roller coaster with me and doing your part even when you don't want to. But I don't tell him these things, I just say thank you again and start to cry.

"Just feel it," he tells me and hugs my head to his chest.

It feels good and still and real.

But I can't stay long.

8

People tell you good things happen when you least expect them. They are the same annoyos who tell you you'll get pregnant if you just relax.

I have to admit, I have been one of these people before I knew better. I have also sought their counsel, especially when I was twenty-five and had barely survived one of those destructive relationships you can only afford to have once in your life. I had crawled back to my hometown, moved in with my mom and stepdad and substitute taught by day and worked in a grocery store at night and on weekends. It felt like some kind of self imposed get-it-together act, a time to stay busy and lick wounds and steep in a familiar nest until I could remember my voice and actually start to hear it again.

It wasn't long until I started noticing men when I'd be stocking the produce, or five o'clock shadowed men near the dairy case, or overgrown surfer boys with wide shoulders and tan hands and flannel shirts headed to the exotic beer aisle.

So I worried. Would I find it? Ever find the real deal? Ever find the one?

"There is no one," Mom said.

"What?" This was news. Depressing news.

"You just find what works."

"What works? That's it? That's the secret of lifelong partnership? Where's the magic in that?"

"Or you just trade them in every ten years. Get a new model," Mom said and laughed.

Okay, I thought, but consider the source. Mom had been through one divorce and remarriage and had, as a marriage counselor, seen the uglies. "By the time they get to me, one person is usually done with the relationship," Mom had explained. "They just use the counseling as a way to break up."

Nice.

But then she would backpedal or try to p.r. the hell out of the "what works" paradigm. "That doesn't mean you don't love each other. It's a friendship. A deep respect."

Oh, god, sign me up! Sounds neato! Can't wait to begin!

I didn't buy it. I knew it could work, but I wanted something that felt a little larger somehow, something with a little more mystery, something with a little more fate. And I just felt in my deepest deeps that it was possible, that I could and would find my soul mate.

But how? How and when and where? And what did I need to do to speed things along?

According to the world, nothing. There was nothing I

could do. I spoke with friends, coworkers, a middle-aged couple at a happy hour bar; they all echoed the same chorus: "It happens when you least expect it."

It seemed so easy for them to say, and they seemed to like saying it, fingers hooked in each other's belt loops, mouths tweaked to the side. It was a secret society of those who had already found their person in the somehows and somewheres of life. I was not a part of it, but I desperately wanted to be.

It happens when you least expect it.

Does that mean I can sit inside my house day after day counting cats through the window because one day my door will ring? Does that mean I do nothing?

So I tried, tried to stop seeking advice, tried to stop thinking about it. I said hello to a man in the bagel store and started humming "We're on the Upward Trail" to derail the impending thought: Can he be the one? But the more I tried to stop, the more the thoughts came. Oo, a smile from the guy buying mango hard candies—potential? Maybe the Rumi-reading-sweatered-man sipping chai? The slouchy-jeans-wearing man with the basset hound? Scuba man? Biking man? Squinty-eyed smoking man? Man whizzing by on rollerblades? No, not that man. But all of them, or nearly all of them, were could be's, and I just wanted to skip the bullshit and get to forever already.

But every one of these thoughts was a step back. I was supposed to not care; I was supposed to be so woozy-woozy-tree-in-the-wind or leaf-in-the-breeze that I didn't get sweaty palms counting back change to Mr. I-Have-a-Nice-Smile-and-it-Shows.

"No, you are just supposed to be into what you are doing," Mom said, stretching her neck out on the word you. "What about your life? Focus on your life."

Obviously I was letting down Ms. Nineteenth Amendment.

I got a full-time teaching job, and while that felt good, it just didn't cut it. I wanted that other thing, the thing I was supposed to be forgetting about.

So I dated Mr. Safety—a divorcé nine years older than I who had a three-year-old daughter and confessed while we sat on a sandy white dune that his wife had left him because she thought he was boring. He was. So I dated Mr. Party—a slim-hipped nineteen-year-old who worked the 2-10 shift at Kinko's so he could drink cases of Natty Ice, smoke pot, drop E and still have time to practice theoretical music mixing on one turn table. He was planning on buying a second as soon as he had enough dough. When I told him he had done well after he had mixed music at an open jam night at a local bar, I had apparently killed our chances. He had faded a song too soon, or scratched a beat too hard, and I, in missing this, obviously had no interest, talent or regard for what it was he was trying to do. Sadly, it was he, not I, who first asked the question, "Tracy, what are you doing with me?"

I started my teaching job and got serious about finding the one. No more extremes, time to find the right person with whom to share my life. Time to be responsible. Find another teacher maybe. That could be a good life. Summers off. Get involved with the community. Never have enough money to buy a house. "Yeah, but after you both have worked a while" (like twenty years), Mom had said. "Look at Jim and me." Mom taught women's studies at the local community college and her husband had taught middle school science for two decades. They had been able to buy a house, but they had bought right before the market exploded. "Besides, owning a home isn't everything," Mom tossed in. She apparently really wanted me to meet a teacher. Maybe she, too, had lost faith in the "when you least expect it" campaign. Maybe I could make it happen.

I tried. I wanted it to happen so badly. I dated, moved in with and got engaged to a teacher. It was exactly how it was supposed to be. Except that it wasn't. It didn't feel right. This wasn't the person and ours wasn't the relationship I had imagined. I couldn't do forever this way. And I was trying for forever. One year later, Mom helped me pack my stuff, and I was so relieved when I saw the note he had left on the coffee table next to the small velvet box. "RING?" it said. Finally, I could stop lying to myself, to him, to the world. I pulled off the ring and liked the way my empty finger looked as we drove to my new apartment. Never again. It's not worth it, I told myself. Never again.

I bought a cookbook and a futon and a queen-sized bed. I volunteered at a dive shop and tried to grow herbs. I'd call Mom every Friday evening.

"You guys doing Nerd Night?"

"Jim, we doing Nerd Night?" I'd hear her ask, pulling the phone away from her face. "Come over."

I'd get my book and walk the four blocks to their house. Mom would sit in her rocker with her book in her lap while Jim would lie on the couch with a paperback three inches from his nose. I'd take the floor and get lost in Orcs and the heaviness of Golum's ring. And by March, I decided to join the Peace Corps.

During spring break I drove to a nearby university to attend a Peace Corps informational meeting. I left feeling unsure but told myself I needed this. If not now, when? Besides, you tried to go to Europe alone and you came home early because you were lonely. Who comes home from Europe early?

The next day I needed to spend time in my classroom. I was halfway down my apartment stairs when I decided to change my sweater. I walked back up the stairs, unlocked the door and found my old college sweatshirt.

On the way to school I pulled over at a copy store. I parked my Jeep in the middle of the slanted lot. I grabbed the handouts I planned on using in my class the following week and got out of the car.

"Get out of the way!" A bald man in a light blue shirt was yelling. Was he yelling at me? "Get out of the way!"

I stepped toward him. He was still yelling. I kept stepping. He kept yelling. His hand went up and pointed.

I turned around and looked up toward the gas station sitting at the top of the lot.

A maroon Eurovan was rolling, rolling; it had been at a pump, but now it was rolling. The gas nozzle was still pushed in the tank and the thick black hose that had ripped free from the pump was swaying, swaying dumb toward the rear bumper. The van was picking up speed.

"Oh-la-lo!" A curly-haired man in a white buttoned shirt was yelling and chasing the van with both arms waving and the black window-washing squeegee still in one hand.

What's it going to hit?

I remember how slowly my head turned on my neck, turned in the same direction of this flat-faced tank gathering its quiet momentum.

My Jeep. My Jeep parked exactly square to the van's path. My Jeep with its one payment left. My Jeep looking so cute there and dumb, white with its black boxy grill, so unaware that it was about to—

I don't remember the noise. It must have been loud. But I just remember seeing the front of the van disappear.

I was light and giddy, thick tongued. Holy shit. I could see the blue of the man's shirt; he was next to me saying something. I nodded. I walked to my Jeep, to the curly-haired man bent over now, his hands on his knees, the end of the squeegee drip-dripping a small puddle by his left toe. He looked up, his glasses were the kind that tint in the sun, and he straightened and wiped his forehead with his rolled-up cuff.

"Is this your car?"

"It's my car," I said, but it came out slow.

There was glass everywhere and the front seat was arced by the roof of the Jeep, but it wasn't until the man had started the van and put it in reverse that I saw just how badly my Jeep had been creamed. The entire driver's side door was pushed to the center of the car.

Through all the events that followed: calling insurance, talking to the police, hearing the thick accent of the man, who turned out to be a French physicist in town for a conference, saying, "But eh had eet een paak!" I really only had one thought—I would have been dead, only seconds off. Fumbling for a pen in the glove box? Dead. Picking a seed from my teeth in the rearview? Dead. Forget the fact that I only had one more payment; forget that it was spring break and now I had this mess to deal with. The message was clear: Be glad you're alive.

"Who do you want to tow it?" my insurance man, whose office was across the street, asked.

"I don't know. Anyone, doesn't matter."

"I'll call Rino's Shell."

When the man at the body shop came into the street and said, "It's totaled. I don't have room for it." I looked at my tow driver.

"What do I do?"

"I'll bring it to the station. If you pay the owner you can probably leave it there."

Anything. I'll pay anything, I felt, quickly realizing that a totaled car is like the dog poop on the sidewalk no one wants responsibility for.

"Can I use your phone?" I asked once the owner said I could leave it there for forty bucks a day.

"It's in the garage," my driver said.

I called my stepdad and hung up and turned around.

"Hi."

Where did he come from? He was tall and thin with brown hair and brown eyes and a one-piece mechanic's suit pulled over his wide shoulders. He was wiping his hands on a rag and looking at me, right in my eyes. Wow. Cute.

"Hi," I said and smiled and walked around the corner of the building to my Jeep. I leaned in the passenger door and knew I should take things, but what? I pushed around the glass. Pulled some tapes from the glove box.

"You go to UCSD?" I heard someone say behind me.

Ol' brown eyes was in plain clothes and straddling his mountain bike.

"What?"

"Do you go to UCSD?" He pointed to my sweatshirt.

Chad claims he would have talked to me anyway, if I had still been wearing the green sweater I had on before my mood shifted halfway down my apartment stairs.

"Okay, so maybe you would have talked to me," I tell him, "but what if the physicist hadn't have washed his windows? What if I had parked in a different spot? What if my insurance guy had called a different tow company?"

"Was there another tow company?"

"Of course!" I'd roll my eyes. (I had no clue.) "He could have called anyone. But he picked Rino's Shell. He picked exactly where you were working."

"We still would have met."

"You think?"

"Baby," he'd say with a smirk and his palms offering up the obvious. "It was destined."

So for Chad the circumstances seemed less important. What was important was that it had happened and that it was great that ours was the relationship that was meant to be.

But I get lost in the wonderment. While I think our

souls are right and meant to walk the earth together this time around, I am aware of the frailty of it all. I'm mesmerized by the way the outcome depends on so many seemingly insignificant decisions made by ourselves and complete strangers. It's as if, while being made discretely, the greater cosmic math was busy clicking those insignificant decisions to greater sums.

This was our beginning, and maybe it's this that has affected our perspective on having another kid. Shouldn't bringing our child into the world be just as fated? Just as magical? Isn't this the way things are supposed to work—with mystery, and loveliness, and a heaping scoop of je ne sais quoi? And as much as a part of me screams, Yes! And it will be! and believes it, with the passing of so much time, another part of me has peeled away, has started to doubt.

Because you know those people who say good things happen when you least expect it? Well, they're the same fuckers who, in hearing of your aspirations for a pay raise, your goal of law school, your lifelong dream of becoming a professional chainsaw artist, will tell you with no trace of irony or hypocrisy to "make it happen." And you'll swallow it. Like them, you intuit and understand, there are some things you leave to the gods and some things you try to control.

Where does trying to get pregnant fall on this spectrum? Is it about making love, opening the door to a potential soul, and bearing the great mystery of life? Or is it about sperms and eggs and mucus and measurements and injections and pills and peeing on tests? Is it about doing whatever it takes?

Four months was all that passed between breaking my engagement and meeting Chad. Had it been a year, two years, or like the two-and-a-half years we have gone without having a second child, would I have joined the Peace Corps and been trying to speed date Uzbek men? Would I have rented a yak and ridden forty-three miles to an internet café just to see who had winked at me online? Totally. That's exactly what I would have done. As much as I would like to say I would have honored serendipity, I know that with time and time and more time, life becomes a *For Dummies* guide. Outcomes depend on trying to figure out how everything works.

9

i do not slide my way to the bathroom. I do not close the door. I do not pee on a test.

I wait.

My dad and stepmom leave. Chad and I get ready for our vacation. Chad has Thanksgiving week off, and we have reserved a house at the beach. Just us, we have said to each other to justify not going to a larger family gathering. "Maybe this could be our tradition," Chad says, "that we always do Thanksgiving just us."

I like the thought of it. And especially like the thought now. Because the time between being fertile and waiting to bleed is the worst. It's when all things are possible, but I do nothing but keep hoping for that one thing. It's when I become three people. And when I hear their voices.

The first and the loudest is the pessimist. She's a brass tacks middle-aged woman with poly prints stretched over her belly and her battle-axe breasts pointy like the prow of a ship. She smokes and wears a kerchief over her rollers. Merle. If I had to give her a name it would be Merle. And even though she might not exist in real life, she is ever-present in my cast of characters.

Why isn't he answering his cell? she says and inhales, You sure he's not shtupping his secretary?

Merle likes to point out the bad even when things are good. And although this can be annoying, the tradeoff is that she also points out the bad when things might be bad and somehow it feels good.

So maybe you're not pregnant. (I picture her shrugging her round shoulders.) Maybe you spend the rest of your days without another mouth to feed and diapers to change. But so what? You'll get by.

So times like these, times when there is nothing else to do but wait and build walls, this friend, who cuts another person's birthday cake, runs her finger along the knife so she can suck off the stack of frosting, is really a warrior. Her only job is to protect me from falling apart when things don't go my way. She actually believes that this kind of protection can work. And even though her tactics have failed so many times in the past (when, despite her campaigns, I do get my period and feel crestfallen) she never opts to ride the bench. Every cycle she is there redoubling her efforts, cinching her kerchief. This time she comes to me as we drive hours to the beach, and Helena has fallen asleep, and the only noise is the hum of tires on the highway.

Hey, she says and points at me with the two fingers that clamp her Virginia Slims, don't go thinking anything is different this time than all the others. You are not pregnant. You will bleed in two to three days from now. You will be all hopey-hopey, and then you will wipe and see dingy blood and be crushed. You wanna keep living that way? I didn't think so. Go buy yourself some tampons.

Then there's Merle's opposite: Sophie. She's the flighty college roommate who listens to Janis Joplin while lounging in her papasan wearing legwarmers, tights and a long scarf. She doesn't go out on dates but is the person the other girls come home to, the person who gushes and bubbles and asks the easy questions and gives them freshly baked cookies and tucks her feet under her when she sits. Sophie has some sadness in her, but she's hopeful, always hopeful. When Merle falls silent for a few minutes, and we pass a billboard for a Dairy Queen, I hear Sophie.

You never know, she says, this could be it. What's that weird feeling you just had a second ago? That twinge like something was going on down there? Why were your nipples so sore yesterday?

But they're not sore now, you dope! Merle cuts in.

We don't need your negativity right now, Merle, Sophie says. I'll just say one more thing: Wednesday. If you make it through Wednesday and by Thursday you still haven't gotten your period, come back and we'll make tea. We'll talk.

And the final voice does not have a name or a persona; it's too wise and detached for either. It whispers in trees and the smell of the morning, and I lift my head and am reminded of bigger things. Let go, it says without saying. Let go.

But I can't, I cry back to it, I can't let go until I just stop trying. Until it never happens and I just stop trying.

The voice says nothing, but I know it is still there. Listening, or letting me listen to myself.

I'm not ready. I'm not ready for that.

So this is how it goes, this time and all the other times in the past. And despite the beauty of the ocean, the coziness of the vacation house with its wood floors and large windows, I still have a triumvirate of voices in my head. Two romp and argue and canvass my thoughts. And somewhere, in all of it, the only thing that's left, and the thing that I try not to feel because it's uncomfortable but seems the most real, is myself fallen away from these voices of certainty into a hazy unknown. I am drifting and looking and trying to hear, but nothing is solid. I can't touch the chatter. And I can't really touch me.

I am lost.

I am totally lost.

Would getting pregnant really make that change? Or is it just something to point to? Has getting pregnant just become a promise of answers, of certainty, the compass rose, a box checked so I can move forward?

What do you do when you have always in your life pictured things a certain way? And when that way just doesn't come true? Can that happen?

Not long after having the miscarriage eight months ago, Chad and I were visiting his mom and we lay in bed under an open window, and I could hear the shush of wind through high northwest pines. It was dark, camping kind of dark, and the window screen shuddered and my cheeks went cold.

"Is there any part of you that can accept that this may not happen?" Chad asked. He was speaking slowly.

"No."

"And is there any part of you that wonders why? That wonders if there is something about you that keeps you from seeing another way?"

"Apparently that's what you think," I said. "Why don't you just say it instead of posing some sort of bullshit question?"

"It is what I think." The sheets shifted. He propped himself on his elbow. "All this trauma, all your highs and lows, all your angst over it doesn't seem right. Bringing life into the world just shouldn't be like this."

I lay flat, still, with my hands like envelopes on the smooth edge of sheet.

"Are you mad?" Don't be mad. Please don't tell me you can't try anymore.

Don't tell me you want to quit.

"I'm not mad," he said and flopped on his pillow.

Good.

"Yes," he said and rose again on his elbow. "I am mad, sometimes. Here are all of you moms who have one perfectly healthy child, and you're all worked up about why you can't have two. Why two? Is it really worth it? Everything you have been through, we have been through, is it worth it? Why can't you be happy with what we have?"

"I am happy with what we have."

"But you want more."

"I've just always wanted two."

"Why? Why though?"

"I just do. There aren't reasons. I can't list things. If I list things it just smallens it, makes it cheap and all thought out. You can't do that kind of thing when you're talking about another life, another creature to love in the way we love Bug. We have two cats. Would I just rather we had one? No, I love both of them. It's the same with another kid. It's just always how I pictured my family. It's just how it's supposed to be."

"But the three of us is beautiful. I just don't know why it's not enough."

"We are beautiful. I know we are beautiful," I said. But you laughed when Helena was born, I thought. Chad cried. "So it's bad that I want another one?"

"It's not bad. I just don't get it. I can get it that that's what you want, but I don't get it for me. And what if it doesn't happen? Can you see it any other way? Can you picture being happy with the family you have?" Chad's arm slid along the sheet. He tugged the blankets. He rolled over. "And if your answer is no, what part of that has to do with you? Take the kid out of it. What's your part in all of it?"

I didn't answer. It was the first time I had spun the camera around. And I didn't hear it until much later, but I think what Chad was really asking was, how far are you going to go? And at what cost?

With two-and-a-half years passed, getting pregnant has taken on its own life. There are times when I don't even think about the child that would come from it, long stretches without any thoughts about the being who would, I guess, have tiny fingers and toes, and its own noises and weight to its bones. But I never forget about trying to get pregnant. I'm not sure if this is out of some self-protection motif, because who really wants to love a child who will never be? Or if it's because I've taken the pregnancy challenge so personally that it has become my proving grounds, something to be hurdled or conquered or challenged and overcome. It has become my nemesis, its own demon, through which I measure my sense of self. Maybe it's just because I've never had my ass kicked like this.

Something about this seems wrong.

But when you get pregnant, that will change, Sophie says and sips from her mug. You'll fall in love with the baby and you'll forget about all of this.

Lighten up, on yourself, Sweetcheeks, Merle adds and leans into her lighter. Anyone would go nuts after all this time.

It's the first time I have heard them agree.

And that third voice? The presence? It is quiet. Quiet and waiting without waiting at all.

I wake Wednesday morning and think, I just have to make it through today without bleeding. Just this one day.

By four p.m. I wipe. Fuck. There is a tinge of brown. Fuck, fuck, fuck. A curtain drops. Everything is flat. I don't want to do anything, but sit frozen and ask it to stop. Don't bleed! Stop bleeding! You are supposed to stay. You are supposed to be here and stay here with me this time.

Chad is in the living room asking Helena which shoes

she wants to wear. We are going to drive to the end of the island and walk down a nature path to a lighthouse. It has been getting windy and the sky is turning grey.

I don't want to go. We are on vacation and this is supposed to be fun family time. But now I'm going to bleed and I want to be alone.

"Pink rapidos," Helena says on the other side of the bathroom door, and I hear her feet thump around the living room looking for them or looking for everything but them.

But I don't feel crampy. I don't feel weight in my back or bowels, or a certainty below my gut. Wipe again.

I'm scared.

Do it, Merle says.

It will be okay, Sophie says.

Nothing.

Maybe it was just the blood that happens with implantation. Didn't you read there can be blood with implantation? Sophie suggests.

When is implantation anyway? Damn, the book is at home.

It's blood, people! Merle says. Just better to accept it now.

I wash my hands and go to the couch. I can just stay here.

Get out in the wind. The thought comes in the whisper of that third voice.

"Did you find your shoes?" I ask Helena.

She brings them to me and I try to put them on her feet. "I want Dada to do it," she tells me. "He's better at doing it."

She pulls the one shoe off half of her foot. She walks into the kitchen, her back straight and shoulders back. "Dada, can you help me with my shoes, please?" I hear her ask.

"Where are your socks?"

"No, Dada, I don't want socks."

"Not even your purple stripes?"

"No Dada, I don't need socks," she says. "Just pink rapidos."

I want to go to a movie. I want to tell Chad, "Let's go to a movie," and have it mean just him and me. I want to hear him say, "Fuuuun!" in a mischievous way and watch his eyes widen at the audacity of going to a movie at four p.m. I want us to bundle up and feel the giggles well up in me big enough that I have to run when we're on the sidewalk which is always his invitation to chase. "I saw you in town this weekend," a student once told me on a Monday. "You were running and some guy was chasing you." I had blushed but laughed and said, "That was just my fiancé." It's not something we plan, but something that just happens when we're together and we're suddenly ten and fifteen and six years old, running just because we can.

"I think we're ready," Chad says.

"Helena, do you have to go pee-pee?" I ask.

"No."

"You should try and go pee-pee before we go."

"I don't want to."

"I know, but it's a good idea to try before leaving," I

start to reach for her.

"But my body's not telling me I have to go," she says.

I am torn between knowing she probably has to go and wanting to honor her decisions so they lead to the natural consequence.

I don't say anything but reach for her down vest and hope she doesn't see me. I don't want to hear how she doesn't want to wear it. I don't want to make choices and have her turn them all down. I don't want her to be so cold when we get there that she says, "No, Mama Bear, I just want to stay here" while she turns her shoulders inward and tries to dig herself into her car seat.

I want things to be easy.

Then why in God's green earth do you want another kid?

I thought Merle was sleeping, but apparently she's not.

You do know what you're signing up for, right? No sleep. Diapers. Swapping who's on duty with which kid. The goddamn diaper bag slipping off your shoulder and everything falling on the sidewalk. It's a pain! And travel? Scuba diving? Where the greenbacks coming from for all that? Where's the time? You think you got grays now!

We load up in the car. We drive until the island goes skinny and we can see water on either side. Chad pulls over and I follow his gaze to a man in a wetsuit standing on the hard brown sand attaching himself to a kite. The wind is blowing against the waves, scudding tops to white spray. The man raises the kite and leans against it while he picks up a surfboard.

"He's going to keep the kite right on the edge until

he's ready to go," Chad tells me, and I can see the kite shuddering, not in full sail.

We all stare. Helena is quiet in the back seat. I wonder if she is okay, but I am scared that if I look at her I will break the spell. She will have an opinion. She will want to unclick from the seat or get out of the car. But she is so quiet. What could she be doing? I slowly turn, just enough to see her out of the corner of my eye. Her head is turned like the rest of us, toward the sea and toward the kite. There is an easy grin on her face.

I look back at the man in the surf. He is on his back in the small breakers, slipping his feet in the straps on the board.

"Watch this," Chad says, and for a second I know he's the one on the board with white foam tumbling around him and wind throbbing his ears. "He'll bring it into the power zone."

The kite dips, and the man shoots out of the water, his black wetsuited body on the white board on the gray waves; he shoots straight and is already getting smaller, like he is headed for the horizon. Like he's never coming back.

"That's so cool," Chad says. He starts the car.

Maybe it would be easier to just have Helena. We could all get back to our other lives. There would be no starting over, just the slow progression towards Helena's independence, which could mean going to the beach while Chad flies a kite, I sketch while Helena reads a book. No more hovering, holding, worrying about wandering off. She could even put on her own sunscreen.

Maybe if it is blood it will be a good thing. Maybe it can be good.

We park the car at the end of the cul-de-sac.

"I have to go poo-poo on the potty!" Helena sings. And even though I know I should do some teaching thing—make her see that it would have been a better choice to have gone at home when I asked her, blah, blah, blah—I don't.

"I'll stay here," I tell Chad who opens his door and steps out in the wind.

I unfold what I call the 007 potty, a portable thing we keep in the car. When she's done, I hold Helena's hand as she jumps from the car. We start to walk.

"Carry me," she says and presses to my legs.

"It's too far."

"No, Mama Bear, carry me," she says leaning enough that I can't move without her falling over.

"No. It's either on my back or in the stroller."

I just want to get to the end of the trail. I know it leads to the sea and a view of an old lighthouse. I want to walk.

"Dada, can you push me in the stroller?" Helena says.

Chad says yes and clicks her in and runs the stroller over speed bumps. She giggles and says, "Faster, Dada, faster!"

He laughs and says, "Again? Nooo." But then takes off running.

You're starting your period. Just accept it.

But it could be something else, couldn't it?

No. You are not pregnant, Merle adds.

Is it bad if I am actually pregnant and you're forcing

me to think negative thoughts? What if that makes me not pregnant? I should be filling myself with light and hope.

Exactly! Sophie says.

Bullshit. You should be filling yourself with truth. You. Are. Not. Pregnant.

The paved path ends at a sandy dune. Chad parks the stroller and unclicks Helena. The three of us walk, Chad and I stopping to wait for Helena. We round the bend and can see the grey green of the ocean, taste the salt.

"Go ahead," Chad tells me. "I'll get Helena." I look at him and want to say thank you but can't. I step around him. "Clear the way for us!" he yells to me as I start walking faster.

The wind bangs against my ears. My body shudders, and the sea keeps beating, and the horizon stays as still as ever, a dark grey line.

Chad and Helena walk the beach as I do but in their own orbit. When they head back up the path, I follow. Chad has already started toward the stroller. Helena is waiting for me at the gap in the dunes. She looks so small there, her little shoulders, her legs disappearing. She looks likes she's coming from the splitting sand, like she's just being born.

"Mama Bear, can you carry me, please?"

I pull her up and feel the weight of her. She burrows her head into my shoulder. "I love you," I whisper into her cold cheek and kiss the side of her head.

"Yeah," she says.

It is Thursday.

No blood.

There wasn't blood Wednesday night and there isn't blood now.

See, Sophie says and smiles and looks up. Maybe it was implantation blood. Just get through today.

But then I hold the toilet paper to the light, and I can see it. A faint trace of brown.

They're called tampons, Merle says and rolls her eyes. She lights another smoke.

But what if—

Tam. Pons. The cigarette bobs in her mouth.

I should. I really should.

It's Friday.

No blood!

Pitiful, Merle says and drops her head and pinches the bridge of her nose.

But there's a chance.

A good chance, Sophie says. You would have bled by now if it was really your period. You saw a faint trace Wednesday. A faint trace Thursday. Today is Friday. Forty-eight hours and you don't have a full-blown period? Like that's normal. Sophie laughs.

I feel light. I don't know why, but I'm dancing.

"Should we bring rain stuff?" Chad asks. He's been shoving things into a backpack, trying to be prepared. We are driving into Charleston today. Leaving the beach to go see the city.

"I don't know, probably," I say as my arms swing wide

and I step my right leg forward. Sheryl Crow is playing on the stereo, and I'm excited to be getting out, excited that we'll be taking a tour of Fort Sumter. My arms come in and I step in and I try to look like a friend I had since I was eleven, Beth. She had signed up for a jazz dance class, and in her black Capezio dance shoes had shown Maria and me her new move. She would point her hands to her pelvis and step one leg back and then step forward and swing her arms wide. She kept at it then, stepping and swinging, until the entire cycle looked like she was plucking hair from her pubis and flinging it to eager fans below. Pluck and fling, pluck and fling, but she'd look serious. This was work. Pluck and fling, pluck and fling, serious shit, serious shit. Add some hip shimmy and Maria and I were mesmerized. "She's good," I had said.

So I do it now, do the pluck, do the thrust, fold in some shimmy and try to look like Beth, eyes forward and mouth closed and so focused I forget to be self-conscious. Every day is in fact a winding road, pluck and fling, pluck and fling, serious shit, serious shit. And it's okay. It's all okay.

"What's up with you?" Chad says laughing at me. "Mama's dancing," he says to Helena who is sitting on the couch staring at me with her mouth like a hyphen.

"I don't know!" I laugh. I am breathless and not stopping. "This dancing just feels good!" And I feel good. I just feel good! "I'm glad we're going over there today," I say letting my arms fall. "I really should know more about the Civil War. It's pretty embarrassing. So much I don't know."

We drive down the island and over the bridge, follow

our map and parallel park at the waterfront. We learn the tour of Fort Sumter will take hours.

"I'll run back to the car and put the quarters in," I tell Chad.

And it's not until I hear the third slip-thunk of my quarter going into the meter that it I hear it. Or I hear Merle.

You're not happy, you dope. And you're definitely not Alex Trebek, 'I'll take Fort Sumter for 400!' Face it, there, Sweetcheeks—

Hope, Sophie cuts in and spoons cereal in her mouth. You're full of hope, she says and wipes her chin.

I don't want to feel it alone. It's too big. I finish dropping the quarters and pull out my phone. I text Tracy, "Still no blood. Keeping my fingers crossed." And I can't help but think of the next text I will be sending her. Pregnant, I'll write. Just one word. I wish I could see her face when she reads it.

The ferry ride to Fort Sumter takes half of an hour. Chad and I laugh at the narrated history they play over the speakers. The voice is the same one from so many movie trailers, rich and buttery and ready to leave you on the edge of a cliff. "The first shots of the (insert sound effects: cannons firing, horses whinnying, whips whipping) CIVIL WAR!"

Chad looks at me and levels his eyes. "It did actually happen, right, the Civil War? Or was it just a winner at Sundance?"

We are the last people off the boat and I stop on the bow to take a few pictures of the sky. The clouds are dark and thick and the water has gone green and shallow looking with white caps.

"That's rain over Charleston," a woman says.

"More than rain," a man says.

The boat staff is hauling out yellow slickers. A bearded old guy pulls on a hat and looks straight off a frozen fish stick meal. He looks cute.

I look back toward the storm that's coming in lines. "Cool," I say. "It's so pretty."

We listen to a ranger and explore the ruins of the battery. It starts drizzling then turns heavy and hits white on the bricks. Chad zips Helena in his jacket. I take pictures.

What an awesome day.

My hand goes to my back. What's that pain?

Rain. Rain and arthritis. Maybe rheumatism. Just a smidge of yellow fever.

We run across the courtyard.

"It's crowded," I say to Chad with my hand on the door to the museum, the only place out of the rain on this side of the fort.

"Can you handle it?" Chad asks. He knows I don't like big crowds.

Today I can handle anything. You might not have heard the news, but I pretty much know I'm pregnant. "Yup!" I tell him and pull open the door.

We read the displays. Helena looks at pictures and counts men in the black-and-white photos. I read, too. Now that I'm pregnant I have the head space for these kinds of things. I read one plaque about a navy ship three times and try to remember names and dates so I can bring them over to my new life. A kind of souvenir of this day. Maybe we'll name the kid Sumter. Fort? Van de Kamp's not too bad.

"Ferry leaves in ten minutes," a ranger calls.

My pants feel wet.

Rain.

Rain! It's wet in your underwear! Merle yells like she's just ripped off duct tape that's been sealing her trap for hours. Enough!

Heavy mucus can be the first sign of pregnancy. Remember what you read online? Sophie says.

Online, don't even get me started with online!

"Is there a bathroom in here?" I ask the ranger.

"There are six on the ferry," he says. "You better use one of those."

I'll know. I'll know in five minutes.

Blood! Merle yells.

Mucus! Sophie counters.

Blood!

Will my hair fall out if they start ripping out each other's? You guys know you're just voices, right?

But why would it come on so strong if it was blood? It does seem sudden. I'm with Sophie on this one. Definitely mucus.

"Mama, can I go with you?" Helena asks, when I tell Chad I need to use the bathroom.

"Sure, you need to go?" I take her hand.

The bathroom is only one large stall. I usually let Helena go first, but this can't wait.

"Mama, what is that?" Helena asks.

I'm staring at the toilet paper in front of me. Staring.

"Is that blood?" she asks.

"Yeah, but I'm okay." I'm okay. I'm okay. It's okay. "You need to go pee-pee?"

"Blood." I text Tracy when we're out of the bathroom.

And it's not until we're back at the beach house that I text her again, "Fort Sumter? The place that started America's bloodiest war, and I go when I'm hoping not to bleed? Smart."

Maybe next cycle I'll take that cemetery tour I've seen posters for. Maybe go skulk around a morgue.

The following morning Chad is standing in the doorway to the kitchen. He reaches to my arm as I walk by.

"You okay?" he says.

He looks at me and I want to say it all and want to say nothing. I want him to ask and don't want him to ask. I want to stop time and rewind and never have to be in this spot with these voices and these stupid hopes and this stupid sorrow eating at me and constantly climbing into my lap. "Just having a tough day."

He pulls me to him and hugs me.

He knows, right? He knows? He knows but he doesn't want to know too much. And you don't want him to know because you might scare him. You'll tip him to the other side just enough that his hands go up in the air and he says he's done. Like the time I went to the ER after I had gone hiking and had wiped with poison oak and had gotten it so badly I couldn't go pee. They were taking so long and I was so uncomfortable and Chad was getting so frustrated because there was nothing he could do, so he had wanted to leave. There is nothing he can do with this either. He has no control and he cannot help and he can't fix any of it, and I can't let him quit.

We're driving back home and I turn around to watch the shadow of Helena's mouse finger puppet on the inside of her door.

"Do you want to go to the beach?" she says in a high voice and the shadow bobs its head as if it's talking and then keeps bobbing when she answers, too.

I turn back around in my seat and watch the flat fields and scrub trees, the way the sky seems to bend it's so big. Will she be one of those kids who talks to her hand and has some imaginary friend who's cute and fun and a completely normal expression of creativity until she goes all redrum on me? Do only-children create these characters more often out of loneliness? Out of a desire to talk to another kid?

I keep watching the road. Chad reaches for my leg and his hand stays. Why isn't this happening? Was it because we didn't have sex the night of our new bed when Dad was visiting? If I had just followed the course of things, if I had let things go how they seemed to be going, we would have made love. And not only would it have actually been making love, but I'd also be pregnant. I'd be sitting here now feeling a whole different thing. What if my uterus is empty all because of not doing it that one time?

Chad squeezes my leg and pats it. "Maybe we should

go somewhere next Thanksgiving. Go somewhere out of the country. Italy or Mexico. Just you, me, and Helena."

Is this supposed to make me smile? Get me all excited and woozy-woozy eyed so I turn to him say, "Really?!"

We are supposed to be in the sleepless throws of a newborn next Thanksgiving! If things go as I hope, we will still be stumbling around bleary-eyed ordering pizza for our Thanksgiving meal. Not traveling! Not flying! Not just us, meaning only us three.

What is he smoking?

Later he tells Helena she is his favorite kid in the whole wide world.

We get home and start unpacking the car.

"Did I do something?" Chad asks out in the driveway. "Is this my fault? Did I do anything to make you so quiet?"

"You didn't mean to."

"What?"

"I just can't deal with the comments. Telling Helena she is your favorite kid, proposing we go to Italy next November. We should be having a kid by next November! We can't get on a plane!" Chad's head is turned. "It's not bad that you said any of that stuff, but it just hurts. It just shows me what's going on in your mind, what your reality is. And the bottom line is, you're not thinking of having a second kid at all! It's like it doesn't even occur to you. And that's all I can think about. We are on two different planets. I hate it."

He hugs me.

"You're right, I don't think about it," he says and steps back. "But I don't really want to think about it. I'm happy with how our family is now. I'm happy with us. If another kid comes along, fine, but I just don't want to work at it, and I definitely don't want to get obsessed with it. The more I see how you are, the less like that I want to be." He puts his hands in his pockets. "But I can try to be more sensitive toward your reality. You're going to have to let me know."

"I was trying to keep you in the dark. I thought that's what you wanted."

"But it doesn't work."

"I get pissed," I say.

"Just keep me in the loop when you're two weeks out. When you think you might be fertile within the next two weeks, let me know. And remind me. And if I forget to ask, it's because I'm forgetting, not because I don't care about you or what you're going through."

"See ya in another thirty-five days," I say and salute limply. And I guess I'm wanting sympathy, a sign that he understands my disappointment at my long cycles that only mean less opportunities per year to get pregnant. But he doesn't say anything. "At least we're on a similar page. I mean what if I were badgering you to do Clomid or IVF and you didn't want to?"

"That would be awful."

"So we have that."

"And we have communication."

Helena is dragging a backpack up the front stoop and trying to open the glass door.

"The thing is…," I say.

"What's the thing?"

"I just feel like in my deepest deeps I know it's going to happen."

"That's the beauty of the mystery," Chad says. "If it's meant to be it will."

And maybe he means something else, but with the words beauty and mystery so close together, I can only see one thing. I will get pregnant. We will have a second child. The mystery will be that it took us so long and that it didn't happen exactly as planned. But the beauty part is that it happens.

10

*t*here's something I haven't told you. Maybe it's because I'm embarrassed, or maybe I just assumed I wouldn't have to. Or I hoped I wouldn't have to because I would get pregnant and I could just leave you with that. But I'm not pregnant, and as much as I'm starting to think it may never happen, I'm ballasted by this secret, this absolutely silly thing.

It's about superstitions. There are many I haven't tried. I haven't gone on a vacation around my fertile week. I haven't gotten wasted with my husband and banged like teenagers in the backseat of the car. I haven't kept old ovulation predictor sticks that say I'm fertile, or slept with pregnancy tests under my pillow. I haven't scheduled a vasectomy for Chad, nor paid anyone to tell me there is no way I will ever get pregnant. I haven't gone to an adoption seminar, looked at foster kids online, or sent for adoption paperwork. I have been tempted to borrow a friend's adoption paperwork, but we decided that in order for it to really count, in order for me to truly reap the cosmic kudos, I'd have to call an agency and order it myself.

Of course the only way I would do this is if I could tell them I didn't want the paperwork but the "paperwork" as if maybe they'd have a separate packet for people who were trying to get pregnant, a packet that directed us to phony informational sessions where we could meet and paw at child actors posing as Haitian refugees so we could make puppy-dog eyes and put pen to paper and realize with a conviction most certain to fool the gods, and nearly good enough to fool ourselves, that we were quite ready to quit the shenanigans of trying to make a kid. Better to give a home to someone who really needs it. Better to not contribute to the planet's growing population. Better go hit the sheets to see if this works!

I haven't tried massaging my nipples, getting a dog, signing up for a triathlon. I haven't committed to a build in Mongolia, looked for jobs, tried sex that involves costumes, handcuffs or leather. I haven't found religion. And I haven't just tried to "forget about it." Because not only am I not capable of not thinking about it, but that idea is just plain scary.

But what I did do?

Eight months ago I called my psychic.

I don't have a hairdresser or a lawn guy, a lawyer, or a mechanic; in fact, I don't even have a dentist. But I have a psychic. Maybe it's because I'd recommend him or maybe it's because I have returned to him three times now in five-year intervals, but his title comes out of my mouth linked with that possessive pronoun we endearingly use with a certain cadre of professionals. It's pretty embarrassing. And doesn't exactly elevate my credibility. But if it makes you feel better, he isn't some brick-ranch-house-on-the-side-of-the-highway-with-a-painted-plywood-sign kind of a psychic. Nor is his name prefaced with Madame or packed with too many j's and t's and k's, exotic looking consonant combinations that must mean he knows something you don't. At worst you might find him at psychic fairs, at best you might find him consulted by police.

Back in April, when Chad's job search was approaching the two-year mark without any leads, we both felt ourselves unraveling with uncertainty. We had wanted to move back to California to get closer to friends and closer to the ocean, but he would send out applications and hear nothing. So one night I said, "Maybe I should call that psychic," as if he were just some dude selling ice cream on a hot day. Although Chad knew I had consulted a psychic in the past, I wasn't sure how he would feel about it now that his issue would be the primary reason for calling. Would he laugh, say I'm nuts, tell me it's like taking a match to a hundred dollar bill?

"Whatever you want to do," he said. "At this point, I don't really care."

He was ambivalent and disheartened, and I could fix all that. I would ask the psychic when and where we could expect to move and while I was at it, slip in a certain other question.

Although the psychic had told me in my two previous sessions that I would have two kids, both girls, I wanted to hear it again. Needed to hear it again. Maybe things had changed, maybe I had stepped off the path and inadvertently killed a butterfly like in the Bradbury story, and the psychic would tell me about my future filled with names I wouldn't recognize and devoid of a second child.

Had I stepped off the path? Had I accidentally fucked up along the way and undone what I thought would be? Like the way Frost knows how things in life go and how it is unlikely that one can return to old places, to old forks in the road. Had I, therefore, taken some turn that had derailed an entire future that was once in play?

Or was it like in those *Choose Your Own Adventure* books? Did you read those? And did you start the book and pick your way through the first set of options, until the robot flies you off to the moon and the book is over on page fifty and then put it down and call the book done? No. Tell me you didn't do that. Please tell me you reread the book, over and over trying out each permutation of choice. Tell me you wedged your fingers in the pages with choices, and tried to read all the outcomes at the same time such that multiple stories were unraveling at once, and that you tried to read like this, flipping back and forth, until you ran out of fingers and the book was too hard to hold.

Does life work that way?

Are there simultaneous realities, whose veracity depends on the kind of reader you are? Are all things possible? Even getting pregnant?

I sat in our car in a Starbucks' parking lot. It was cold out, and I pushed the latte between my legs and hunched over the pen and paper in my lap. It would be getting dark soon. The traffic buzzed on the highway behind me, and cars eased from the drive-thru in front of me with their headlights dipping and scanning the yellow brick building across the street. The two previous times I had appointments with this psychic, I had gone in person. But now that we lived on the other side of the country, I didn't have a choice but to use the phone.

I dialed at the time of my appointment and asked about moving and Chad's job first. Then I got to the goods.

"Am I going to get pregnant?" My voice went high and the phone felt thin and flimsy against the side of my face.

"You just have one child?"

Aren't you the psychic?

Let the man do his thing!

But this is his thing, isn't it?

He's not going to waste his psychic energy on incidentals! Get to the big stuff!

"Yes."

"Oh yeah," he paused and then chuckled. "You're going to have another. You want the good news or the bad news?"

"The bad."

"You're going to have another girl."

Ha, ha, ha. That's funny! That's hilarious! The psychic laughed, too. Wow, is that a hoot!

Phew. It's the same, the same news as before. Nothing had changed in my cosmic recipe; I hadn't chosen the wrong adventure. Apparently everything, including all the time and difficulty we had endured up to that point had been part of it. It had all been meant to be.

"It won't happen until you guys get settled, though. Looks like in about eight to ten months."

It would be December then. December was the month. Latest February. Pregnant by February.

I drove home and was glad to see that Chad had already put Helena to bed. We could talk completely uninterrupted. There was so much I had to tell.

"Apparently you're going to find a job," I had told Chad. "In five months we'll be moving to Southern California."

The psychic had already emailed me an audio copy of our session, (a complimentary service), so I pushed play on the file and let Chad listen to the part about our someday kid. Chad chuckled when the psychic cracked the joke about another girl. I wanted to look at him, laugh with him, but I was trying to play it cool. I stayed looking at the computer and whistled in my head, doo-da-doo, no biggy, just another day of validation that the very thing I have been wanting for forever is going to happen, whistle, whistle, whistle, no big deal.

And guess what? We had moved in five months. The psychic had been spot on.

Chad had found a job and we had moved in exactly five months.

Where? Why are you asking where? Sure, we had wanted California and the psychic had said Southern California, but that part doesn't really matter, does it?

Okay, okay, South Carolina, Chad found a job in South Carolina.

"At least he had the initials right!" I had said to Chad later and laughed and remembered the political cartoon that had shown George W with big ears and a pointy nose circling the Q's in Iraq and al-Qaeda.

But all hope is not lost. He's just a temporal psychic, and timing here is all that matters. Who cares where I get pregnant? He said eight to ten months. Some time between December and February.

That's what I've been holding onto. Through the moving and the unpacking, through the traveling and the house guests, through the tests and not using tests, through the disappointments of blood, what the psychic said just confirms what I already know to be true. Call it intuition, call it a hunch, call it that deep knowing inside. I felt it before I met Chad. I knew I would meet a true lifelong partner, and look how that turned out. Sometimes you just know.

Latest February, maybe even before.

11

i slide out of bed and run my feet across the floor like skating. I shut the bathroom door. I sit on the toilet and wait for my eyes to adjust to the glow of our nightlight. I open the drawer. Pull out test. Tear foil wrapper. Click test into holder. Pee. Pee. Pee more. Pee on hand. Recap stick. Tear off toilet paper. Wipe holder. Place test in drawer. Close drawer. Wash hands.

Mission accomplished.

I turn on the light and open the door and wash my face and put on my pajama bottoms. It has only been two weeks since my period ended. Today is probably not the day.

I brush my teeth and put on a shirt. Two minutes down. Time to open the drawer.

Survey says.

O

I eject the stick in the trashcan.

I go downstairs.

Later that evening I am sitting on the floor with Helena. Chad is somewhere in the house, maybe on the computer. It's Christmas time, and I asked Chad to bring the red and green Tupperware bins down from the attic. He did, then he disappeared.

"What's this one, Mama Bear?" Helena asks pulling at the ball of tissue paper in her hand.

"I don't know, unwrap it."

This is supposed to be fun.

I spent the morning at the art store gathering supplies to make our Christmas village complete: snow, garland, a little girl figurine for Helena, a boy flying a kite for Chad. Even though we don't have a rug and a couch and there is nothing hanging on the walls, and even though we will be spending the actual holiday with family in Kentucky, I want our house to be cozy.

It's a pretty low bar really, but one of my biggest priorities as a mom is coziness. I want Helena to have coziness. When we first moved in I even trawled Craigslist until I found a man selling a double papasan chair.

"You're kidding," Chad had said. "Those are so '80s. '70s even. Guys in the navy had those things."

"I know, but they're cozy."

"And ugly."

"It's only for the back porch," I had said.

It's one of my favorite ways to spend mornings with Helena when it's cold. "Go get some books," I tell her. "I'll get the blankets and meet you in the nest." On really good days our orange cat comes in the nest, too.

Helena may have other resentments someday; I can

picture a twelve-year-old version of her coming to me and saying, "Mom, no one wants to pick me in PE because I can't shoot a basket."

And I'll say, "But what'd they say about the track suit I made you, huh? Fleece-lined? Down stuffing? Pockets on the legs for all your friends."

"But, Mom, I can't throw a ball!"

"Who needs sports, Silly, when you have a track suit that holds all of your friends? Look, kitty-cat can go right there in the pocket on the thigh. And monkey? How bout monkey? Don't you just feel all snuggly and good?"

She may never learn long division or learn how to write her name, but at least Helena will have cozy. She must have cozy.

I lay the snow in the fireplace we have never used, even pull off a section and drape it over the log grate to make it look like a snowy hill. I have already unwrapped the village candy store. A leafless tree. The mirror that's supposed to look like a frozen pond.

"It's the man," Helena says and she drops the tissue paper and holds the little figurine to her face. "The man with something. What is this, Mama Bear?"

I lean over. "An accordion," I say. "He must go with the singing girl."

This is an odd village handed down to us by an old neighbor who had moved and insisted we take all his decorations. Even though he had lived alone for many years, he had boxes and boxes of decorations: strands of lights and glass beads, cookie tins, ribbons new and used, Muppet babies with Santa hats, bears stuffed and hard, a

Santa whose hand you pressed so he would say, "Remember, the magic of Christmas lies in your heart." He had a plastic tree, reams of tissue paper, stacks of cards, felt banners, candles, a nutcracker whose mouth didn't open tall enough for a nut. We told him we would never use everything, but he told us that we must, that we had to take it all for the sake of the baby. He had always called Helena "the baby" even when she was walking and running and asking him where his cat was and why he had shaved his beard. So we had taken it all.

Last Christmas we had put together the plastic tree and set up the village for the first time. "It's so cute," I had said to Chad when we made the room dark. The lights on the tree glowed, and the chips of light through the village windows had made it seem like little people were really living inside.

"Pretty cozy," Chad had said.

We had stared for a while feeling something. Responsibility? Gratitude? Nostalgia?

And here we are again. In front of the same stuff. And another year gone.

"He goes here," Helena says and tries to push the man in the snow. He tips. I pull the snow to make a hole and she tries again. The man stands with his back to the house that is on the hill and is much too large to be lived in by a single person. He stands looking over rooftops below with an accordion draped between his hands. He is looking at nothing. Looking at something. Waiting. Or playing on a snowy hill into the night.

Something is missing.

"You know what we need, kiddo? That dog. That black and white one. Do we still have it?"

"This doesn't work, Mama Bear." Helena says and holds up a lamppost whose battery pack swings from two skinny wires.

This stuff is crap. Complete made-in-China crap. But our neighbor had tended to it, had returned each piece to its original box or rolled it up in tissue paper and taped the edge. He had also taken a Sharpie and labeled each one—Candy Store '07, Skating Pond '06, Choir Girl '08. I'm not sure if the date was for the sake of reminiscence (it's not like the village was going to spoil) or for some kind of Dewey Decimalesque categorization. But after a few times of going into his house I had begun to notice it everywhere—Push Broom 03/07, Eby's food 08/09, Dijon 09/09. "Have you noticed the dates on everything?" I asked Chad one time. "Why do you think that is?"

"It's just Bob," he said and smiled. And I had liked that answer, that sometimes there aren't reasons for things; we just are the way we are.

But something about it seems sad now, as I sit in this dim room, pulling hand-me-down holiday detritus marked with Bob's writing from this plastic bin and unroll the thin white paper gone wrinkled and soft.

Something is missing.

The clock radio had glowed amber. I had watched a six turn to a seven. My brother had whispered, "You awake?"

"Yeah," I had said. It was 11:38.

We were at my dad's house. He lived in an apartment,

and my brother and I shared a room at one end of the hall. I slept on the lower bunk and think I would have picked it anyway, even if my brother didn't always pick the top.

But sometimes being on bottom was bad, when B'd do that thing with his arm. I'd be about to fall asleep and the arm would appear, hanging straight and dead from the top bunk, straight down with fingers limply curled. I would see it there and say in a regular voice, "B, I know you're awake." But he wouldn't say anything. And the arm would just stay. "Yeah, right," I'd say and try to turn my head in the pillow and go to sleep. But I couldn't sleep, not with that thing hanging so straight and lifeless like it was something unto itself, some dead and has-been creature crawled from the crypt. Hanging. Just hanging.

"B!" I'd say, lowering my voice. Maybe he had just fallen asleep and his arm had rolled off. Maybe something had happened. "B?"

I'd start for it, not wanting to, but having to, one finger reaching from my covers, reaching up. I'd touch it. Touch the side of his hand with my finger and pull my hand back. Nothing. Just his hand.

So I'd touch it again and again until I was pushing it and the whole arm was swinging and settling, swinging and settling, swinging and settling back straight.

"Come on, B," I'd say, but he was quiet. No noise, just the arm.

I'd try again, pushing and thinking if I just pushed it hard enough, enough to make it hit the edge of the bunk, it would disappear. But it didn't. There was only one ending.

I'd reach and push, reach and push, reach and push,

rea—grab!

It would grab me. The silent hang-dead hand would be alive and strong and grabbing my wrist.

I'd yell.

My brother would laugh.

I'd say, "I hate when you do that!"

And he'd say, "What'd you think?"

And I'd say, "I thought you were dead. I didn't like it."

"From how it swung, or what?"

"And how it just hung there."

"What'd you think at first?" he'd say. "When you first saw it?"

And we'd go on debriefing and I'd love talking to him in this way, back on the same side and being consulted. I'd like hearing him laugh quietly at my narration of thoughts or hearing him make a noise that meant he was smiling. Of course I was just giving him more data to perfect his routine, but I'd never remember that the next time it happened. There would always just be the arm and me reaching for it, and the grab and the scream and the anger gone soft the minute we were friends again.

But on that night before Christmas, he just whispered down, "You awake?"

"Yeah," I said.

"You excited?" he said.

"Yeah. Don't do the arm, kay?"

"I'm not doing the arm."

"Not the whole night though, okay? Not just right now but later, too," I said.

"Turn on the radio," he said.

"But seriously," I said.

"Okay. But turn on the radio."

"I don't want to get out," I said.

"You're closer," he said.

"Not really, I'm just lower."

"I'm way up here. Come on."

So I pulled back the covers and went for the glowing lights. 11:41.

"Where's the button?" I asked.

"On the side."

"Close your eyes, I have to turn on the light."

"Don't turn on the light!"

Finally I found the right knob in the dark and with a click and a hum we had music, some kind of violins and a man with a library voice, thick and deep between songs.

I know we talked about presents, noises coming from the living room, whether or not Santa would eat the cookies even though we both knew Santa wasn't real. We talked about snow and sledding and moon boots. And he said, "Didn't they used to smell or something?"

And I said, "They'd smell because we'd leave that inside part on the heater and it would melt. And they'd stain our socks, remember?"

"That's right," he said and I knew he hadn't remembered until I had said it, so I felt like the keeper of things. Always the keeper of the tiny things as if it were my duty. We talked in half sentences and long pauses like the way you think to yourself or talk straight to the night.

A little past 1:00 there had been a cooking show.

Near 1:37 I had said, "You take-a zee cheeken..." imitating the guy on the radio.

"That's pretty good, T," my brother had said. "That's pretty good."

I take the lamp from Helena's hand and try the switch. Nothing happens. I wiggle the wires. Nothing. "I'll go get new batteries."

When I come back, I stop in the dining room and am aware of the cool weight of AAs in my hand. I look at Helena who is still sitting on the floor with so many fluffs of white paper around her that she looks like a small island. She is holding something close to her face and talking to it in a high voice that's the voice of pretend.

And then I see her. The other one. A dark, curly-haired girl with gapped teeth and a loud smile. A girl who sits cross-legged with her hands reached around to her toes. A girl who does not unwrap the contents of the Tupperware bin, but makes jokes and silly faces and who wants Helena to look. She is sitting there rocking up toward her knees and back to her bottom. She is sitting on the bare part of the floor. She turns to me and smiles.

Come.

Please.

Come.

"The doggy, Mama Bear," Helena says. She holds up the thing she has been talking to in her hands. "I found him."

"Cool, kiddo," I say and walk toward her. "Now our village is complete."

But I wonder if I can ever mean it. Mean it if it's just us.

12

i slide out of bed and run my feet across the floor like skating. I shut the bathroom door. I sit on the toilet and wait for my eyes to adjust to the glow of our nightlight. I open the drawer. Pull out test. Tear foil wrapper. Click test into holder. Pee. Pee. Pee more. Pee on hand. Recap stick. Tear off toilet paper. Wipe holder. Place test in drawer. Close drawer. Wash hands.

Mission accomplished.

I turn on the light and open the door and wash my face and put on my pajama bottoms.

If today is the day I'm screwed. How will I ever get Chad in the sack after eight hours of driving? How will we do it in the squeaky bed at Grandma's house?

I brush my teeth and put on a shirt. Two minutes down. Time to open the drawer.

Survey says!

O

I eject the stick in the trashcan. Hey stick, I say in my head like the stick is a telepathic speaker phone and I can send direct transmissions to my ovaries or to whoever it is that's running this show, I'm not saying I'd be unhappy if you did decide today is the day. I mean, I'll take anything; I'll make it work. But today is just not the best day, that's all. But tomorrow? Tomorrow's fine. We can do tomorrow. Or any other day. You just give me that smile, okay? I'll take care of the rest.

I lay one square of toilet paper over the plastic, but leave the peed on part sticking out. It looks like it's being tucked in.

Chad finishes packing the car, and we pull away from the house later than I would like, but we should still make Grandma's by dinner. Hours later the road is wet and black and winding between mountains close and rocky on either side. I think we're in Tennessee. The heater is on; Helena's asleep. I touch the glass of my window; it's cold. My dad and stepmom will be at Grandma's, too. With their dog. At least they brought the baby gates, so the idea is to keep Helena and the dog apart. I hope it works. I hope everything works.

"You know," I say to Chad without turning my head, "how we talked about 'give you a heads up' and all that?"

"About what?" Chad says with half a smile. He's got his vacation aura on, which means he grins a lot and leans back in chairs and lets his hair go shaggy and his stubble grow. I like his vacation self, so I'll forgive him for not knowing what I'm talking about.

"About the pregnancy deal. When I'm fertile."

"Yes, that," he says and puts his other hand on the steering wheel.

"It should be any day now. I have the sticks with me, so I'll keep testing. But we may have to do it at Grandma's. And that bed."

"Whatever it takes," Chad says and smiles. He looks at me. Puts his hand on my knee.

"We may have to do it on the floor," I say.

"I'm on board. Whatever we need to do." He pats my knee. Puts his hand back on the wheel. He's quiet.

But he's my teammate, my shipmate. And at least this way I'm not standing behind the curtain in Emerald City trying to come up with things to give the Tin Man and the lion with those hideous curls.

"Can I go into Grandma's room?" Helena whispers and my ear goes hot and wet with her breath. She's in bed between Chad and me. Somewhere in the dark morning, she stood up from her mattress on the floor and climbed in between us.

"She's not up yet," I say. "Try to sleep." I roll over. In fact, no one in the house is up yet. This may be a good time.

I pull the Ziploc from my suitcase and open our bedroom door. The hall is dark except for the small lamp at the top of the stairs and the nightlights plugged in on either side of the bathroom mirror. The floor creaks three times. I pass the room where my stepmom is sleeping. My dad is downstairs on a blowup mattress with the dog. I hear the clink of her metal collar. She is awake and shaking her head. Or she is standing up. I close the bathroom door and lock it. I wedge the iron loon doorstop behind it just in case the lock breaks. I pull out the test. Tear foil wrapper. Click test into holder. Pee. Pee. Pee more. Pee on hand. Recap stick. Tear off toilet paper. Wipe holder. Place test on counter. Wash hands.

Mission accomplished.

I wash my face and brush my teeth. I read the labels of three small French soaps that are on the back of the toilet. I open the mirror of the medicine cabinet. Bottles and creams and pill jars. Excuse me. I feel like I have interrupted something. I close the mirror. I sit. I will just sit. I will sit still like a non-snooping, respectable, non-interloping house guest. No peeping Toms here. Doo-da-doo.

The hour glass is still turning on the test. It's processing. Is it bad luck if I just stare at it?

I look away. I look back.

O

Oh.

Okay, test, but tomorrow. Tomorrow.

I look at the trashcan. Since this is the only bathroom upstairs thus used by nearly everyone in the house, the can is nearly full with typical bathroom bric-a-brac: fluffs of Kleenex, Q-tips, an empty box of pink Dove. How bout I just fling the ovulation test right on top? And just see what happens. No doubt it would be disturbing for someone, like the time I saw a friend's dad's colostomy bag hanging in the shower. It's not like I had known what it was, but I didn't need to. Something about the plastic and the dangling straps and it being in the shower had alerted my senses to the far-too-intimate. It was a thing for a body, not a person, but a body, as if the two were suddenly separate, and with its unfamiliarity, it had also been a sign that something was not normal. Something was, in fact, wrong.

I do a double tug of toilet paper so the strip is three feet long. I wind it around the test. And just when I think this is a good enough cover, I picture five days' worth of mummified sticks. The news is bound to get out: Come one! Come all! New Egyptian mouse exhibit happening right now in the baby blue trashcan! Seniors get in free! And if that happens, someone's going to get all curious and pull a loose tab of the toilet paper until the whole mess unrolls and the sticks plink on the floor. And regardless of whatever sense one makes of the contraption, there will end up being kitchen-whispering and elbow-nudging and a suggestion that everyone except for Chad and Tracy go make a trek to the corner ice cream joint for sixteen-scoop sundaes even though outside it's fifteen below. With all their good intentions, people will want to tend to us, to the jacked-up couple, who just can't seem to get pregnant.

I shove the used test in the Ziploc with the holder and the other tests. I walk back to our room and open the door. Chad is sitting on the edge of the bed in jeans and a t-shirt. He's putting on his socks.

"Everything okay?" he says.

"Yeah. Not today. You're off the hook," I say and hold up the bag.

He smiles. I stuff the bag in the underwear section of my suitcase.

The next day: O
Oh.

O
Come on, already.

O
You've got to be kidding.

O
Fuck.

On the drive home it's dark when we're in the mountains. It starts to snow. Chad slows down. The car is warm and still has the new car kind of smell. The snow in the headlights falls fast and quiet. We're quiet, too. Maybe this is better; I'll be fertile when we get home. We can actually do it in our own bed.

I slide out of bed and run my feet across the floor like skating. I push the bathroom door. I sit on the toilet and wait for my eyes to adjust to the glow of our nightlight. I open the drawer. Pull out test. Tear foil wrapper. Click test into holder. Pee. Pee. Pee more. Pee on hand. Recap stick. Tear off toilet paper. Wipe holder. Place test in drawer. Close drawer. Today for sure will be the day.

I wipe. Something's dark.
I flip on the light. I sit and wipe again.
Blood.
How can that be?

I open the drawer.

○

I never ovulated?

My body just decided to sit this one out? Ride the bench?

I snap the test in two pieces. I shove each one in opposite sides of the trash.

Chad pushes open the door that I hadn't closed all the way.

"You okay?" he says.

"I just got my period."

"Oh."

"I never ovulated."

"How do you know?"

"All the tests. The little fucking test. I did them at Grandma's and everything. I've never been fertile."

Chad hugs me.

"I'm sorry," he says.

"Mama, look what Bear is doing," Helena says as I pass by her door.

"I can't, kiddo." I go downstairs.

One of my friends told me you can tell non-fertile cycles by a lighter amount of bleeding, but by later that afternoon, I know she is wrong.

Every time I change my tampon, chunks fall out. I used to call them livers because they reminded me of what I had seen my mom bring home from the deli maybe twice a year. They were pink chunks in a puddle of dark blood, and she'd fry them with onions and the house would smell and I'd wonder how she could eat such a thing.

The period livers also used to gross me out. Actually when I first started getting my period, they scared me. I can remember standing in the shower and feeling something and hearing it slap the tub near my feet. I wondered if something was wrong. I must have asked someone, probably my stepmom who was nonchalant about these sorts of questions. "It's just part of the uterine lining," I'm sure she would have said. Maybe she's even the one who first called them livers. I don't know anymore. I just know once I knew it was normal, I liked being the first in my group of friends to say, "I've got total livs today" so I could hear them say, "Oh" like they had just been socked in the gut. They were grossed out, too, but they'd use the word themselves until the shuttling of the word and the reaction felt like it brought us closer, like our bodies were bringing us closer to each other, closer to ourselves.

But today I hate my body.

I've been hating it all day.

"C'mon, kiddo," I say and walk to Helena's room and take a book out of her hand. She is sitting on a large plastic bus that is an old toy she is too big for, but that she had spotted when I had pulled down the attic ladder to find a suitcase for Kentucky.

"Mama, can I have that, please?" she had asked standing at the base of the ladder. I had tried to play dumb.

"What?"

"That," she had said pointing. "The bus Mima and Grandpa gave me."

I had wanted to say no because I wasn't sure if it would

start a monsoon of old toys and clothes and books being pulled out of the attic. Maybe she'd want to play in her exersaucer or Jonny Jump Up or want to sit in her highchair for her meals. Maybe she'd want to revisit *Baby Says Peekaboo* whose pages were torn and edges bitten or take baths in her duck-hammocked bathtub. Because it is all there. Our attic is stuffed with all the things I have kept. Orange bins and pink bins and clear bins with tape marked 0-3M fall, 3-6M winter and on and on. Shoes and books and receiving blankets we never even used. "Just think of the money we'll save," I say to Chad every time he complains about the attic getting full. "We'll have to buy diapers and wipes next time, but we already have everything else." Chad usually just looks away.

"Okay," I had told Helena that time before Kentucky, and now here she is on the bus with her legs splayed out like bridge cables running to her stripe-socked feet.

"I was reading that," she says when she sees me put her book under my arm.

"I know, we can take it with us," I say.

"What are we going to do?"

"We have to go to the store, come on."

"Why the store?" she says and flings her head over the steering wheel. Honka-honka! Her forehead hits the horn. She looks up, her mouth round, and then she laughs.

"Come on, kiddo. You need to put on shoes." I reach for her body and try to pull. I lift. The bus comes, too. "Hey!" I say. I put her back on her feet.

"What?" One of her hands is still on the blue steering wheel even though the bus lay on its side like a wreck.

"We have to go. You need shoes. No bus."

"What do we have to get?"

"Milk," I say. "We need milk."

"I don't want to go."

"If you don't walk downstairs and get your shoes on, I will carry you down."

"I can do it myself."

I load her in the car. It's grey outside, the kind of winter grey that's really white and undecided. Scraggly trees. Black road. We drive and see five cars in a row that are white or silver. At the stoplight I watch the cars' yellow blinkers tick together for a second. And fall out of sync.

What is wrong with me? The tissue, all the blood. That should be someone's warm and dark place to grow, someone's nest, but it's just falling, falling and settling in a black pile at the bottom of a toilet bowl. What a waste.

The light flicks green.

"Mama, why do we have to go to the store?"

"Milk."

But it's not for milk. And it's not even for ovulation predictor sticks or pregnancy tests. This is for something else. I know the store will have them because the store is a chain. And this is around the same time I got them last year. But last year I was alone.

We need milk, too.

"I want to walk," Helena says when we get to the sliding doors and she sees the green carts.

"Stay close to me." I take an arm basket.

The music is fancy. Fancy and lacy and smart like someone else's life. The lights are dim and glowy and the fruit shine-shiny and the vegetables burst in their green dampness ready to urge me to health and a perfect life with the perfect smell, the perfect noise, and all the perfect choices laid out just so. Just choose. Just pluck. Just look at your list and point a finger and say, "Not that one, too pink, that one, please." And tell them no, at the deli, when they ask if it's okay if they cut a little too much. Say no, I'd like two pounds. Two pounds on the nose. And tell them you want it thinner. Tell them you want it shaved. Tell them to start all over again. Get exactly what you want.

"You having fun with Mommy today?" a woman behind the cake case asks. She has long graying hair pulled in a bun and her lipstick is pink and slick. She works here and her head is peering over the domed case looking at Helena.

"Yes," Helena says and leans into my leg. I stand dumb and look at Helena, too. I don't want to talk. But I won't have to. This is the part when they ask her how old she is or they tell her they like her hair or her shoes or, because she's a girl, tell her how pretty she is or ask her if she is a princess.

"It's just you and Mommy?" the woman says and puts her arms on the top of the case so she can lean further. "No brothers or sisters?"

You've got to be kidding.

"No," Helena says.

The music is going from some speakers in the ceiling. The strings swell. The woman's forehead is wrinkling. Her top pink lip is coming to a point in the center. I want to smash her face into the cakes.

"No brothers or sisters?" she says again but looks at me with her chin receding into her white collared neck.

"Nope," I say.

Forget the cakes. I'll smash her face into the case.

"Well, that's fun!" she says and turns to Helena with a wide pink smile splitting over her white teeth. "Just you and Mommy out together. How fun! I could never do that because my mommy always worked. You're a lucky little girl!"

You've got to be fucking kidding.

I pull Helena's hand. She holds up her free hand to wave.

"Can I get a cookie?" Helena says looking at the case with its trays and racks and rows.

How can people just ask that stuff? Just say that stuff?

"Just one," I say. "But we split it. You pick."

"Chocolate chip," she says.

"Pull out a bag. They're over there."

"Can I carry it?"

"Okay, but no eating until we buy it."

"Mama, milk!" Helena points to the corner we have passed.

"That's right. Thanks for remembering."

That's why we came. Why we came here to this store five miles away when milk is sold on the corner two blocks from our house.

The milk slides to one end of the basket and bumps against my hip. Where are they? Cheese popcorn sounds good, too. Don't they have them? It's after Christmas, but they should still have them. They have to have them. There is an endcap of cookies, blue bags and red bags, bags with stars and frosted trees. Those are good, but they aren't what I'm after. I want those circles, those puffy circles with their Euro-spiced dough and German name and thin skin of frosting and chocolate that your teeth tick through on their way to soft goodness. I want them on their sides, stacked and cellophaned and calling out, "Fresh from the Hinterland! Exotic! Limited time, now!" I want the confidence of the dough, the memory of the spice, the neatness of the trim paper tray that slides from the plastic wrap. They're by the checkout! I squeeze Helena's hand. Maybe I'll just have one this time. Okay, maybe two.

"Can I have my cookie now?" Helena asks when we leave the register.

"No, kiddo. Wait till the car. We'll eat in the car."

I see our car in the treeless lot. Steam rises out of a shiny pipe from a roof across the street. It blends with the white sky. Just get to the car. I strap Helena into her seat, start the car and turn on the heat. Someone has parked in front of us. A red SUV has pulled its nose to ours. There is a man at the wheel. A man with sunglasses looking down. Is he reading? Just waiting? Why'd he have to pick this spot? Will he know what I'm doing if I leave?

"Okay, kiddo. We're sharing, remember?"

I reach back and take the half she has broken for me, put half in my mouth and open the bag of cheese popcorn and slip the bag between my leg and the door. I pull the plastic string on the spice cookies, slide them out and place them on my lap, close to my stomach.

"Kinda bright," I say and shove a cookie from the tray

into my mouth while I'm hunched over my purse digging for my glasses. I chew. It's much too big, but I chew some more. Another. I need another. Bite. Bite and chew. Hmmmmmmmmm. The humming starts. It's loud. Loud in my head. Popcorn. Bite and chew. Hmmmmmmmmmm. Bite. More. Bite and chew. Blue dumpster at the end of the lot. A trash can in front of the store.

When I was sixteen, maybe seventeen we had been in the car, too. I remember it was the car because we weren't looking at each other. Mom had asked me, "So when will you consider yourself a woman? I mean do you think of yourself as a woman now?"

I don't know if it was a change in her voice, that it was a hint louder or more clear, or the way the question would seem apropos of nothing, but I knew this was not serious talk or a personal thing. It was some kind of data collection. Maybe she had just read some study, gone to a conference or had some discussion in her class. But this was some kind of litmus test, and for some reason it made me feel important. Or relevant.

And you know what I thought of first when she asked? My period. Did I have my period? I had never seen anyone in real life say, like those after-school-special moms, "Congratulations, you are now a woman" when the daughter had gotten her period, but that criterion must have seeped in my bones. This criterion whose assumption I didn't realize until now: you are woman because you can have children.

But that's wrong, I had thought at the time. I had started

my period, and all it meant was that I had to get my cat to sit on my uterus to help ease cramps, that I had to worry every time I stood up in class that I had bled through my jeans, and that I still couldn't find time for a tampon change between Algebra II and French. The whole period thing definitely did not equate to womanhood.

What about sex? I hadn't done it yet, so I couldn't say. But I could see it like a math problem: penis + vagina = womanhood. It just didn't feel right.

"No," I told mom. "I don't think of myself as a woman."

"When then?" she had asked and started to grin.

I had paused, but not too long. It was pretty easy. "When I can support myself. When I live alone and can pay all my bills and maybe even buy myself some shoes."

God, it had been so easy. It had been so clear. I suck the cheese off my index finger. Bite and chew. Time for a cookie. One more. Or maybe one and one and one and one. Shove. How can I shove them all in? Just keep stuffing. Stuff them in.

"Mama, what are you eating?"

"Hm?"

"What are you eating?"

It had been so easy to see what a woman was. But what did I know then, sitting in a car and seventeen? I had everything in front of me, assumptions I didn't even know I had.

"Mama!"

I take a piece of popcorn. Hold it to the backseat.

"Yucky, I don't much like it."

Does she know? Can she see my hand go to my mouth

back and forth and back and forth? I reach for her book, the one from home and put it in her lap. I open it to her favorite page with the cat. Don't look at me. Cat. Look at the cat.

"Oh, I like him!" she says.

I run a handful of corn along my side. Just shove. And now thirty-seven and this: dying eggs, barren, infertile, eggs that are drying up. I have a woman's body without a woman's function. I am a failure. A failure who deserves to be parked in this lot with a running car and a child strapped in back; a failure who has earned the sneaking, hiding, shoving, stuffing and the frantic and the humming head and the hand that knows what to do.

Eat. Just eat.

But I want to hit. I want to yell. I want to kick myself and watch my body, this growing soft body with its boobs too small and its thighs too big curl on itself and go small. I want to kick myself and watch the fat jiggle. So I can hate. So I can hate more.

No brothers and sisters? And the way she had looked at me. Like I was cruel. Like it was my fault. And Helena just answering the question. No, she had said so plainly. No.

Three left. Just get it done.

When I was in college I bought a box of Thin Mints from the Girl Scouts who were selling cookies on campus. I walked home with the box shoved in the pocket of my canvas coat. I opened a roll and walked and ate. I ate whole cookies at a time, pushing them in my mouth, walking and eating while the wind blew and cars rushed and my feet scuffed on the hardened dirt of an empty lot. It was midday and Tracy, who had been my roommate, wouldn't be home. I kept eating. Something in my head was loud and I could feel my hand lifting the flap of my pocket again and again, chipping off another cookie from the crinkly roll.

By the time I got home six cookies were left. I put down my backpack. I took off my coat. The bathroom was dark except for the light from my bedroom window cutting long shadows from the right. I knelt in front of the toilet and shoved my finger down my throat. I gagged but knew if I really meant it, I'd have to shove it farther. I shoved. I gagged. Don't have what this takes either. What a fuckup. I cried slumped over the seat. When I straightened I could see my face in the mirror, puffy and round and cut off at the neck by the back of the toilet. The captain of the varsity rowing team. The face of a leader, right here.

Do something different.

Do something different.

I look up. The man in the SUV is looking up, too. Fuck you. Are you looking at me? Fuck you. Fuck you and your waiting and your dark sunglasses and your fucked up choice in parking spots. Fuck you, and whatever you think you know. You don't know me. Fuck you.

My hands fall. White crumbs cover my lap, the seatbelt. There are even some on my sleeve. I kept telling people, "Why bother?" When I'd talk to other moms about the loose plate of skin that stayed at my belly after Helena was born. After it stayed and I ran and ran a half-marathon and went to spin classes and it still just hung and filled in with fat. "I just figure, why bother," I'd say and laugh. "Why bother when I'm going to have another one and just have to lose it all over again?" They had laughed too and understood. It had all made perfect sense. And it's still here, here hanging over the seatbelt.

But it's fat. Not fat with a promise, not fat like a chrysalis. Just fat.

I'm scared.

I am so scared.

"Mama, are you sad?"

"I don't know," I say. "I'm okay." I take the plastic bag and fill it, fill it with what's left. A rolled bag of popcorn. A cellophane wrapper. An edge of one cookie rattling in its stupid tray. I stuff it in and cinch the handles. The bag poofs like a stomach, bloated and long since drowned.

"Can we go home?" Helena asks.

"Yeah, kiddo. I'm done. I'm done." I pull out from the spot and pull up to the curb and throw the bag away in the pretty green garbage can in front of the store.

13

*d*o you ever have a memory that comes to you again and again like a reoccurring dream? It's the kind of memory that loops through you while you're jogging or about to cross a street or that flashes suddenly when you see a woman run her tongue over her teeth before she pulls open a restaurant door. It's the kind of memory that seems to come out of nowhere, but starts coming and coming often.

Two days ago I was pushing Helena on a swing, and just as I felt my fingers slip from the cold metal triangles at the edges of the swing's seat and watched Helena's head dip and rise as her feet came out in front of her, it came to me again—Dena from sophomore health class, her voice like she had just drunk milk and hadn't cleared her throat.

"Oh, God, look at Mr. G's dong," she had said and rolled her eyes, like the thing in our teacher's pants was throwing spit balls at her or raising its hand too much.

But then she grinned. She, too, had shifty wonderings but not first-hand knowledge of that thing that bulged the fronts of pants. But pants of an old guy, though? That was gross. And disturbing.

Sophomore health was a class that had already made me uncomfortable in the way it had lacked the familiar. There weren't desks to offer some island of security or justification for sitting alone. This class was held in a corner of a sprawling cafeteria with fluorescent lights and rows of tables and a guy in a jumpsuit steering a mop and pushing a yellow bucket with his shin. And there were too many faces that looked in compact mirrors and smacked frosty lips before the bell rang or faces that needed to shave their chins or swipey-swipey that hazy film that had settled in the fronts of their eyes. These were the upperclassmen, and it was implied by the way they slumped and clustered at the ends of the long tables, that it was the class, because it was so dumb, that had failed them, instead of the other way around. So they'd say nothing, or chuckle, or cough to cover the word "bullshit," and raise their hands only when they wanted to go to the bathroom or to debunk the presented stats.

"That's not what happened when I smoked pot," one might say, and our tenth-grade eyes would swivel to the kid, to Mr. G, to the kid. "I didn't get hallucinations; it was great."

A few kids would say "humph" in their hands or "ch" and look down, but most of us stayed pale-faced and slit-mouthed, watching and waiting, assuming swift death, silencing, or at least dismissal to befall the mohawked kid or the shaved-head kid or the girl with flannel shirt and ripped jeans who was out of nowhere alert and leaning.

"Okay, okay, class," Mr. G would say even though no rowdiness had ensued but instead silence, that hungry and anxious silence that spreads quickly and teeters on what teenagers will make of the world. "Heroin is a narcotic," Mr. G would continue, tacking to the heavies to minimize the chance of personal narratives and thereby increase the ease of his stance. He'd keep reading his Xeroxed stats with his feet apart and his hips pushed forward while he rocked to the fronts of his toes.

Health class was full of this stuff—following "along on the sheet in front of you," looking "on with your neighbor." There were worksheets and handouts and bookmarks with numbers to call if you felt like blowing out your brains. And maybe the superficiality of bits of paper and taking notes was an attempt to lighten the weight of every topic that always led to certain death. Smoking? LUNG CANCER! Drinking? CIRRHOSIS! Smoking a jay? DROWNING IN TWELVE INCHES OF WATER BECAUSE YOU FORGOT TO STAND UP! Or maybe it was the only way to teach stuff that we certainly couldn't do. If Mr. G had said, "Today in sex education Sam will roll a condom onto his penis and put it in Sally's vagina," he probably would have gotten a few calls.

However, the simplicity of phone numbers and dittos and guest speakers who, as part of their parole, gave talks on how steroid use leads to ax murdering, left out all shades of grey. Did every person using steroids end up zit-backed and throwing their girlfriend down stairs?

What about all the times a kid could drink before ending up with a liver like sopped bread in a bus-line puddle? How about all the kids who had smoked pot and still made the honor roll? What about all the adults whose cars were full of Whopper boxes, loose packs of Kools, and a case of Milwaukee's finest in the trunk, while having jobs and spouses and children?

It didn't add up. But I was fifteen, and it was enough to have these questions. It was enough to untie these knots without squinting at the pieces of newly-humped cord and tracing them to their frayed and messy ends. Messy ends would come later. At fifteen I was inexperienced, so I swallowed the health curriculum whole. Even when that thing in Mr.G's pants continued fuzzing straight lines.

The first time Dena had pointed it out, she had leaned in and I could smell the chemical sweet of hairspray on her double roll of bangs and thinly feathered sides. Dena and I were class friends and hall friends, the kind of friends who find each other out of the desperation of not knowing anyone else.

"Look," she had said from one side of her mouth.

I had followed her eyes to Mr. G who was in another typical stance: foot up on the seat under the cafeteria table, forearms leaning on his bent knee while his hands rolled the sheets of paper, let them loose, folded them like a taco, rolled them again. He'd listen this way and look like an old guy caricature—tinted glasses, black hair as sprayed as Dena's, taupe skin and taupe v-neck golf sweater pulled snugly over a polo shirt. He always wore some kind of coordinating polyester pant and shined pointy shoes. He definitely checked the mirror in the morning, no doubt lingering to smooth stray hairs, sprits cologne and pat his abdomen before stepping outside. He was also older than my father, and barring any greasy-headed comb-over man with eyes in two directions, I pretty much trusted any man who looked like he had kids or grandkids and kept a bat in the closet to bash in the heads of people attempting them harm. Something about Mr. G was safe but sad.

Which was exactly why I had no idea what Dena had been trying to show me.

She turned so I could see her face straight on. She leveled her eyes, and her lips stretched over her teeth that though small seemed to make her mouth hard to close. "Down there."

I'm not sure how old I was when I first learned it, but I was well versed on the meaning of "down there." Down there has only ever meant and will only ever mean one place.

My face twisted as revulsion hit. Not Mr. G. One of those wide-shouldered, narrow-hipped juniors? Maybe I would have been happy or at least curious to look at the front of their 501s because, thus far, my understanding of the penis was limited to a few strange and accidentally collected data points.

When I was ten I saw a bouncing pink something when my father, who had run from the shower to the living room to catch a Marine Corps commercial on TV, had leapt up from behind the couch, fist in air and shouted, "Hoo-rah!"

At eleven, I had been de-icing a fruit punch flavored

Big Stick by running my hand up and down it quickly when my brother's friend saw and chuckled.

"What?" I had asked him.

He laughed more until he finally said, "Do you know what you're doing?"

"Getting the ice off," I said.

"You look like you're doing something else."

I can't remember what he said next exactly, but whatever it was, it had led up to words I will never forget: "Then white stuff comes out."

"White stuff?!" I had said and had looked at my brother who snapped his eyes from a far-off gaze.

"Dude, that's enough."

"Yeah, white stuff."

"What do you mean?"

"Dude, I'm serious," my brother had said and sat up on the couch. He had been serious, and his friend had shut up.

Of course I had raced to the phone that night. "Beth, white stuff comes out!" This was hot-off-the-press serious shit, the kind of shit whose passing along was not only urgent and required in friendships, but the kind of thing I hoped would get passed then pinned to me. Maybe the popular girls didn't know about the white stuff yet, and didn't that matter? Shouldn't there be a tally being kept and a few points hashed to my name?

That was seventh grade. In eighth grade sex-ed the mystery was cleared up when we learned about ejaculation. So that's the white stuff! I had thought, glad for the knowledge but also bummed. (So much for getting a head start on cool.)

Nonetheless, the penis continued to be an enigma.

During a dance that year, lights low, "Penny Lover" playing in the background, Nancy Pew told five of us girls that when she had danced with Aaron Z, she had felt his thing swaying to the beat of the music.

"What do you mean?" we asked. Nancy closed her mouth and raised her index finger. We squeezed in shoulder to shoulder, watching and breathing in sync while her skinny finger bent up and down, up and down, like a curling periscope, in perfect time with the harmonica solo. I was so confused. I was confused by her use of "swaying" to describe vertical motion. And I was confused that the penis had talents, or maybe just Aaron's penis had talents. Do all penises keep time?

Dena was still waiting for me to check out Mr. G's crotch. I pushed my eyebrows together, pleading. Do I have to?

"Tracy. Look," she whispered.

Using my name and using her vocal chords? Dena was upping the ante. I rolled my eyes and took a deep breath.

At first I didn't see anything. His foot was still propped on the seat of the table so his knee bent at ninety degrees and the material of his fitted pants stretched in long thin rolls from the top of his thigh to his bottom of his zipper. And sure there was a roll in his zipper where it was folding onto itself, but that even happened in my jeans when I sat. Relieved, I started to turn to Dena to tell her she might want to stop snorting lines of marijuana before class.

But then I saw it.

That's why Dena's eyes kept going ping-pong balls.

"No," I whispered. "That can't be—"

"His dong," Dena mouthed and her eyes went big again and her lips hung round so that even in silence I could hear the g in dong rubberbanding on itself. Why'd she have to say it like that?

I looked back at Mr. G's crotch. I looked to the right of his zipper and let my eyes fall along the inner seam of his straight leg where his pants, because of his bent leg, were pulled tight. There, for about six inches along his inner thigh, was a bulge the shape of a banana or sausage or French baguette. Maybe he had strapped a sandwich to his inner thigh? Yelled to the missus, "Fix up a hoagie!" while he pulled a sandwich-strapping contraption up his hairy leg like it was just another tube sock? Had he poured soup in a condom and kept it there for warmth? There was definitely a bulge, and it was so perfectly shaped I could practically see the schematic of his silhouette with a dotted line pushing out from his thigh and filled with the words "Insert penis here."

"Does he know?" I asked Dena.

Dena rolled her eyes.

"No, does he know we can see it?" I asked.

"He wants us to see it," Dena said from behind her fist.

What? How can that be? An old guy, a guy older than my dad, somewhere in that hazy zone, too old to be my dad but not old enough to be my granddad was teaching at a school with teenage girls and wants them to see the outline of his obviously large dong? Or worse, the shape of his obviously large pretend dong?

Weird.

And not only weird, but hypocritical. Why flash your dong when you're up there telling us it's the very path to death or paralysis or the hander-outer of seeping sores on various pink and shiny-skinned parts of the body or the potential transmitter of "cauliflower-like warts"? Because even more than the booze and drug portion of the curriculum, the whole intercourse deal was fraught with landmines. If it wasn't enough to be afraid of having pustules oozing out of your privates, there was always AIDS. Or even worse, the big P word.

At that time, AIDS still seemed remote enough, a disease saved for headlines, whereas pregnancy was for hallways. It made the news between classes when the throng of teenage heads bobbed and shuffled and laughed and called and notes were passed and hands were shaken or slapped or held limply and shoved deeply in the pockets of jeans. Pregnancy was real because if nothing else there were pregnant girls in the hallways, too, laughing loudly and pushing a friend's shoulder and busting out the Aqua Net behind the flaps of their locker doors. And pregnancy was also real because even though condoms seemed much more apt to be used than dental dams (has anyone ever even seen a dental dam except for in the scissored fingers of a milky-faced guest speaker?), and even though the condom's ninety-eight percent success rate seemed pretty high, there was always fear. "Think about it," Mr. G would say, "would you want to be that two percent?" or "What if the condom breaks?" or "What if it's not put on correctly?" or "Condoms have been known to come off inside the woman and the sperm leaks out and GOES EVERYWHERE!"

It wasn't like Mr. G was preachy or scary or trying to lecture with these statements; he had been around a little too much for that. He was a facts guy: present the facts, and if we balked, he could always rely on one of these questions and ask it in a rhetorical way. "What if the condom has a hole in it?" he might say and put up his hands and tilt his head to the side like he hated to be the bearer of bad news, but that hey, my friend, condoms have holes. And until seeing his ginormous penis, I half way, no, actually full way believed that Mr. G spoke the truth. Sex means pregnancy. And even after factoring in the hypocrisy of his dong billboard, I still believed it: Every time you have sex (barring the ninety-eight percent who used condoms and are just plain lucky) you get pregnant.

I maintained this belief despite even more evidence to the contrary. Mr. G rolled in the TV cart and pushed play on a video that showed real sperm being ejaculated into the vagina. It was that one video that was like an Indiana Jones movie as thousands of spermatozoa get annihilated in the vagina's "hostile environment." The squirming cloud is finally whittled down to one rather Harrison Ford-esque spermatozoon who out-swims and outwits his delirious brothers who suffer defunct tails or get snared in vaginal folds. I remember being vaguely struck by the apparent odyssey the sperm had endured and how that contradicted the if-you-even-think-about-sex-without-wearing-a-helmet-you'll-get-pregnant notion. But that thought was derailed by a more immediate concern.

The hostile environment of the vagina.

Did they have to say it like that? Already the vagina seemed like such a mixed bag. Somehow I had intuited that a lot of boys wanted their penises in vaginas. But then there was that other notion. The one I had witnessed in the bus line when Heather Johnson crouched on the sidewalk to repack the books that had fallen out of her backpack, and some dark-haired skinny kid had stepped out from the back of the line and said, "Close your legs! It smells like fish." I had wanted to die. And as much as there was another me in another life who wanted to turn and tell the kid to shut up, the me in the bus line only felt scared. I, too, was Heather Johnson, and how quickly he could turn on my privates. But was it true, boys wanted vagina and were repulsed by vagina? Or boys wanted pussy, but were repulsed by vagina? It was yet again confusing. And watching thousands of happy, squiggling sperm go stone dead in the hostile environment of the vagina probably wasn't doing wonders for the vagina's already sketchy rep.

So that's what I held onto. At fifteen I was so worried about the vagina's p.r. that I didn't actually let what I saw on the screen sink in.

But that's all I keep thinking about now.

The mass destruction, the obliteration, the absolute stone cold dying of so many potential little half-lives keeps rising from the depths of health class at age fifteen. At fifteen, enough seeped past my insecurities such that I saw the gap between the statistical wasteland happening on the screen and Mr. G's warnings about pregnancy. But

I stowed that gap as a feeling, a fuzzy feeling shoved in a bag of contradictions, which is why the video memory is also paired with the thing in Mr. G's pants and the assumption that teachers didn't have penises or shouldn't have penises or at least shouldn't be warning us about sex if they were going to fling their giant dongs around. But in the past several weeks, and days ago, while I watched Helena bob and rise on the swing, this memory comes, rising to the surface and blooping open like a sea-bubble yielding to sky, and nothing about the contents is fuzzy or paired with anything else. It stands alone. And it's clear.

You idiot.

I see the video cart with the TV strapped on top and our dark and tiny silhouettes reflected in the glass. Mr. G pushes play and a cloud of sperm blooms and tails squiggle-squiggle and heads wiggle-wiggle as they silently call and swim and exalt. And I want to name them all: James! Natasha! Vladamir! Marcus! Hey, check out Bachita!

But they die. Hundreds die. Millions die.

Possibilities are snuffed again, again, again.

Until.

There.

Is.

One.

One tiny one winning the golden egg.

It was there. At fifteen, I just didn't see it, but the truth of my current reality was there, staring me in the face.

Getting pregnant may not be easy.

I should have known. I should have seen! Mr. G should have said something! Why didn't he say anything?

I'm on my way home after dropping Helena off. I drive by a crossing guard who stands on the corner in a neon vest and waves with a neon-gloved hand. I hear Dena, "Oh, God, look at Mr. G's dong." I let the memory play. We're in the cafeteria with Dena and Mr. G, and the video is playing and the cloud of sperm is filling the screen.

I stop the memory. I push pause somehow and start painting different events, hypothetical events.

Mr. G pushes stop on the VCR. He clears his throat and holds up his palms. "I know you aren't thinking of this now, folks," he says, "and it is true that if you hold hands with each other while you are teenagers, you will probably get pregnant. But it is also true that if you wait too long, if you actually wait until you're thirty-seven, you won't be able to get pregnant at all! AT ALL!"

My brain pans to my fifteen-year-old self in her acid-washed jeans and her poofy bangs. Would I be staring with my mouth agape? Would I be frantically scribbling with a quivering hand 37!! with circles and boxes and arrows around it and a skull and crossbones inked over the digits?

No.

I wouldn't even be looking at Mr. G. I'd be doodling in the margins, drawing his pants in ways I could quickly convert into squirrels or large-nosed sheep. Tell it to someone else, I'd be thinking. Me, at thirty-seven? By thirty-seven I'd already have two kids and a house and be making yearly jaunts to the Cote d'Azur. That's what I'd be thinking.

So I can't blame him. I can't even blame the fifteen-year-old me for letting her own insecurities about penises and vaginas and her own naiveté keep her from tugging at the nagging contradiction on the video screen and keep her from realizing (based on the strange goings-on in Mr. G's pants) that things are not and probably won't be what they seem. But I can look at my expectations: By thirty-seven I will already have two kids.

This thought, and the certainty with which it was cemented in the vision of my future, would have alone prevented me from hearing any caveats Mr. G could have said. Without me even realizing it, the thought was determining what information was relevant and what was not, and in this filter-like way, it kept and would have kept me from considering any other way my life might go.

I can still see the edge of the crossing guard's vest in my rearview mirror. I see her tiny bright hand wave to someone else. I look back to the road in front of me, wet and drying in patches where sun is coming over trees.

Are all expectations like blinders? What's right in front of me now that I just can't see?

14

*i*t's half way through January. Mom and Jim have come for a visit. They have been here seven days and are about to leave; they're only doing a final trip through the house to see if they've forgotten anything. I catch my mom in Helena's bathroom while she gathers her brush and scans the shelves. She says something to me, and I respond with the comment that's an obvious invitation: "Maybe that's why I'm not getting pregnant."

The whole time they have been here I have wanted to talk about it but I haven't. What is there to say? Is it possible for my mom to listen to that conflicted ball of so many words and so much silence as a friend, devoid of her own interests in having another grandchild? Is it even fair to ask her to do that?

But without planning it or even thinking about it, this bait flops from my mouth. She's standing in the door of the bathroom, and I'm standing in front of the sink. With five minutes left in their visit I bring it up? Why?

"Well, you're going to try for another year, aren't you?" Mom responds.

That's why.

There is something flat and calm inside me. Without knowing it, I baited her so I can practice saying it, this calm and new thing I'm starting to feel come true. I want to tell someone else so I can hear myself say it out loud and use the float of words to seal the deal. And I want to let any interested parties know, they are on their own.

"Not for another year. I'm getting ready to give up."

I am not shaky or big-eyed. My voice doesn't come up like I'm asking a question. But as I say it I'm not sure if "giving up" can ever sound true or if it will only ever sound sad, pitiful, a handful of hurt teetering on yes or no, finalities born of desperation and hopes dashed, not from time peeling from time. "I think we'll keep trying until June."

She just looks at me and pulls her mouth to a line. There's no more to say.

I slide out of bed and run my feet across the floor like skating. I shut the bathroom door. I sit on the toilet and wait for my eyes to adjust to the glow of our nightlight. I open the drawer. Pull out test. Tear foil wrapper. Click test into holder. Pee. Pee. Pee more. Pee on hand. Recap stick. Tear off toilet paper. Wipe holder. Place test in drawer. Close drawer. Wash hands.

Mission accomplished.

I turn on the light and open the door and wash my face and put on my pajama bottoms.

Today might be the day. It's February. This is the month the psychic said. This is the month it is supposed to be. And just in case not everything rides on psychics or supposed to be's, Chad is taking those sperm-boosting vitamins. When Mom had gotten back to her house, she called and told me that forty percent of the time infertility is caused by an issue with the man. I had read that before, but done nothing about it, so this time I did some research and lined up three different pills for Chad to take twice a day. Just in case. Talk about having our bases covered.

I brush my teeth and put on a shirt. Two minutes down. Time to open the drawer.

Survey says!

O

I eject the test and hold one end with two fingers over the trash can like one of those claw machines in a Denny's waiting area. I open my fingers. The test dives in the can.

I leave the bathroom. Chad is sitting on his side of the bed.

"This is going to be a bad one," he says and turns to me. I know he's not talking about a cold or a hurricane or the next set of waves rolling in. "You have to let me know."

"Bad because we're trying so hard?" I say. "Or bad when it doesn't happen?"

We're having two conversations at once or we are in two places at once, both before and after the event.

"Yes," he says and reaches out to me.

There is one answer to both questions.

I sit next to him. His shirt is still open. His belt dangles from its loops. "I'm going to get busy with work and I don't want you to think 'Oh he's not asking because he doesn't care.' Just let me know if you get your period or something."

"Okay," I say. "I really appreciate you being so involved."

But it's February. And it's different this time.

"And you have your vitamins to take," I say and smile and don't want it to sound like I'm nagging. "I wonder what will happen. What if you end up with enormous balls?"

"I'll be sitting at work at my desk and suddenly," Chad says and makes a sound that's half explosion, half Batman comic. His hands flare wide.

"Boulder balls," I say.

"Just call me Boulder Balls."

We laugh.

And I want to remember this. Laughing. Us. If we end up with another child, if we end up with one child, our relationship is what will be left constant and changed and standing. The steady beat of our navigation and building of each other is what will last. And what will matter.

But not as much as another kid will matter!

It's still there. The other voice. The voice that's growing frantic and loud as if it knows it may one day be snuffed out.

It has to happen this month! It's meant to happen this month! Remember the psychic said eight to ten months! Ten months is February! February is now!

Even though we're being open, I don't tell Chad about this part. I don't want my added expectations, the number of times February is circled in red Sharpie on my mental calendar, to mess things up.

"It'll be okay," I say and stand up.

15

*t*hey are back. Everything went as planned: I got the smiley face, we had sex on exactly the right days, so now I'm waiting. And they're back.

You're pregnant, Sophie says and sucks on the end of her spoon.

I can't believe you're even letting her in here, Merle says. Merle wipes her forehead with the back of her hand.

But your boobs ache. Sophie holds up a finger. And you haven't bled yet.

Why does your back ache then?

You went on that bike ride yesterday. Maybe it's that.

It was six miles! Merle lights a cigarette. And completely flat!

It is day twelve of what I think should be a thirteen day luteal phase. Twenty-four more hours of wonder, doubt, agony, foolishness. Twenty-four more hours of incessant banter: You're pregnant... No you're not, you idiot! This is what you thought the last time! Go eat some ice cream! It will calm your nerves! Or try pancakes this time!

And just how many times am I going to go check my underwear for blood? I now have a bring-it-on tactic. It's like when I was a kid and after seeing the movie *Psycho* had spent the next twenty-seven months flinging back shower curtains any time I'd use a bathroom. It didn't matter that in the movie the victim was in the shower, and it's not like I had a plan for what to do were I to find a thin man with a wig on standing in there with a butcher knife, but I couldn't stand the fear, the not knowing, all the what-ifs growing and burbling behind the hang-dead shower curtain while I unzipped my pants. I had to beat the fear. Race it. Know better. And it's the same now. Every time I go to the bathroom and feel a waver of fear, I wipe aggressively and quickly. I zing it around. Snake eyes, motherfucker! Stick 'em up! Check that white paper, home dawg! In that moment after the zinging I'm like one of those bad horror movie combinations, but instead of *Jason vs. Alien* I'm Billy the Kid meets Snoop Dog. I'm shoving a six-shooter in the side of lurking blood; I'm trying to bust a cap on my own period before it busts a cap in me.

I'm losing it. My crotch will be raw by the end of the week. What am I doing to myself?

I'm not sure what I'll do.

What will I do if I bleed?

But it's different this time. It's February. The psychic said latest February; now here it is.

And if it doesn't happen?

It will happen.

What will I ever have to go on?
It will happen.

That night Chad and I are in bed. I stare at the lines the blinds make across the window. They hum. They scratch and zig. I can't keep my eyes still. I open them farther, try to bug them and hold them still. I turn them to the ceiling.

"I think I'm going crazy," I say. But it's not a crazy voice at all, but stiff and still, everything my eyes can't be. "Just so you know." The person speaking is somewhere else. I know her but don't know her; she is far away behind so many smooth walls.

Chad doesn't say anything. I look at the cats, black silhouettes against a dim blue darkness. Our fat tabby pushes my hand.

"How are you feeling?" Chad's voice comes measured and slow and clear enough to mean he has been awake.

Is he feeling my heaviness thunk on his chest just as he thinks his day is done? Is he rolling his eyes in the dark? Does he dread this conversation?

"I'm fine," I say. "I shouldn't have brought it up. It's dumb."

"Why are you saying that?"

"Because I'm not sure you really want to know."

"I hate that. It's not giving me any credit. It's not fair to me."

It's easier to write about it, to tell everything to an imaginary reader, a sister who's going through the same experience than to share everything, every fear with my best friend and biggest stakeholder in this process. Does he mean it? Can he take it?

"I'm just so tired of the thoughts," I start. I list examples. I tell him about the wiping. I tell him that I've let myself have the thought: I'm pregnant. I tell him I hate myself for it. It's too quiet. "Are you there?"

"Yes."

I continue. Then stop.

"I'm so sorry," he says, but he's small. He sounds unsure, on shaky ground.

"Are you okay?"

"Do you think we have done something wrong?" he asks, and his words come clean without rustling or hands pulling sheets. "I used to think the three of us was a beautiful thing, but now it's like I've listened to you for too long. I see siblings everywhere."

"The three of us will always be beautiful."

I'm a hypocrite. Who am I to try to give this back? I wish I could feel it, feel what I am saying, but I can't. I pull on cold knowledge, but the warmth of any real conviction is gone.

"Should we have tried harder earlier? I didn't know we should be banging every second as soon as Helena was born. Did we do it wrong?" Chad says.

"We couldn't have been any different than we were. We could only do what we thought was right at the time," I say. "There's no point in regretting anything unless we are going to use it to fuel a different decision now."

And I mean this, but I also think I know what he is feeling. I had already dragged myself over the coals of regret with my sophomore health class. But I had also realized that no matter how loud the voice of my thirty-seven-year-old self could have been yelling, "You will not be making yearly jaunts to the Cote d'Azur, and you won't have two kids!! Wake up!" I had accepted that the current pull of my fifteen-year-old truth would have been too strong. I wouldn't have been ready for a different truth. I couldn't have seen things any other way.

And if this is always the case, if at fifteen I knew I would have two kids by thirty-seven, and at thirty-seven I know I will have them by thirty-eight, and by forty I am telling myself, "Guess I was meant to have them by forty-one," then does it mean that I'm just a shitty guesser at truth? Is it that my intuition-detection-unit (that keeps sensing that THIS is going to be the year I am going to get pregnant) just needs to be retooled?

Or does it mean there are no external truths? Does it mean that my intuition about knowing it will happen is actually just my ego putting words to desire and expectations and cloaking them as truths? Does it mean that my sense of it coming to be—my "I just know in my deepest deeps," my vision of our family of four walking down the beach—has all along just been a creation of me and my small brain instead of a large external truth? Does it mean there is no such thing as meant to be?

"I'm sorry I brought it up," I tell Chad.

"Don't be," he says. "I don't want you to feel alone."

"I'm just scared. I'm not sure if I can handle the blood. I'm not sure I can go through all this again. What will I ever have to go on? And how many more times? How many more times can we do this?"

"We'll do it as many times as we have to. We'll do it together." His voice is still thin and his arm doesn't come around me. He doesn't reach for me or touch me in any way. But he is my partner. And even if we are both reading from scripts, from the cue cards of what we know we should say but don't really feel, I know he will always be the one across from me practicing lines.

We lie on our backs like two corpses. I don't speak again. I close my eyes, and the buzzing in my head is too loud to keep them closed. I breathe and look into the dark.

16

*i*t's Friday evening. This morning I woke up feeling a little less afraid. Maybe just because I didn't wake up to blood, or maybe because in talking to Chad last night, nothing was solved, but at least it was shared. But I still spent the day listening to Sophie and Merle.

Why are your boobs sore?

They're not sore. You're imagining things, little Miss Dreamcatcher. Go dance with your scarves!

But you are a little nauseous.

It's called 1600 calories worth of cheesecake! Go buy another Save the Wolves t-shirt!

And as much as Merle was being a little too harsh, I know she is right: It's coming. I know it's coming. It's day thirteen of my luteal phase, so it will be here tomorrow. Maybe even tonight.

After dinner, Chad, Helena and I walk downtown. I hold Helena's hand when the roads are busy. Her cold fingers curl around one of mine and I rub the backs of her fingers with my thumb.

We get to the coffee shop and slump in a corner booth. We take out Helena's markers and she gets busy drawing pigs. Pigs with cat smiles. Pigs with long legs and big feet. Pigs the same size as flowers. Pigs holding hands with ladybugs.

I look up at Chad. "You're staring," I say. He's looking to the right and down a short flight of stairs to another room with tables and chairs. No one is in there except for one young woman sitting in the corner looking plump and pretty in a purple shirt. She folds her lips in and out like she is spreading lipstick. She checks her phone.

"I'm trying to figure it out," he says from the left side of his mouth. He doesn't turn his head.

"What?"

"Why they wanted to sit back there."

"Who?" I ask.

"The woman sitting there is with that guy at the counter. They hugged and he walked her to that room. Now he's getting their coffee."

"Is that room even open?"

"I guess," Chad says, "but why would they want to be there?"

"In the corner, too," I say. "Maybe they're gonna do it."

"And we can watch," Chad says and looks at me with eyebrows raised and mouth still open.

"Ew!" I say. I put my hand on the side of his head like I'm going to push it but I don't. I like Chad's head, his face, the smell of his hair just above his ear. I like him. I like him a lot. "Which one's the guy?"

"That one," Chad says and nods as he takes a sip of his coffee.

I follow the direction of the nod. A young guy is standing at the counter, his back to us and his muscled arms hanging at his sides like parenthesis. He is wearing a white shirt, a white lycra job.

"What's with the shrink wrap?"

"Just pumped some iron," Chad says and hits his chest with a fist. "Feelin' good!" He's in the same voice he used to use after hours of engineering homework when he'd put down his pencil, point and say, "You have to work to be number one!"

"Then why go hide in a back room if you're all about showing the world your pecs?"

"Blind date," Chad says.

"And he's not so stoked on what showed up?" I say and push my back against the chair.

"Baby," he says slowly and raises his eyebrows, "what if people think we're a blind date?"

"And I showed up with my kid. Surprise!"

"What a great surprise," Chad says and looks at Helena. She is still hunched over her paper with her hair dropping around the page. She raises her head but doesn't turn to us, only starts a new pink circle that's dotted with extra ink where she's paused. I sling my arm around Chad's neck and pull him in. I kiss his hair above his ear.

"I have to use the bathroom before we go," I say and stand up. I pass the bulletin board in the hall. I step in the bathroom and turn the lock of the stall door. I don't want to look.

Don't then.

Just this one time, I just want to wipe like a normal person.

I know, so don't.

Just give me this night.

Don't look. Don't.

White.

My shoulders drop.

No fun being a fool, Merle says. It's coming.

Sophie whispers, Maybe you are pregnant this time. Maybe you are.

That's when I think of the poem. Do you remember it? It's the one by Emily Dickinson? The one about hope.

> Hope is the thing with feathers
> That perches in the soul
> And sings the tune--without the words
> And never stops at all...

I keep thinking about it as I walk back to our table, put Helena's markers back in their box, swing the backpack to my shoulder, smile at Chad when I see him looking at me with his eyebrows pushed together. And even now I keep hearing the first stanza in my head as we walk under this sky, sun-sunk and washed thin with wind and slivered with the moon already glowing like a smile.

"Look, kiddo," I say to Helena as Chad hoists her from the sidewalk onto his back. "The moon. It looks like a smile."

It really does. It is a thin crescent but rocked on its back. It's so white and small and perfect it would almost be corny, a corny smile, except that it's the moon.

"Did you see it?" I ask, worried that her head was too smudged in the back of Chad's hood to see.

"The moon, Da-da. It looks like a smile," she says, and even though she's just copying me, it might be the first time she's said a simile. It's what we do, I guess, without even thinking about it we give our children words and structures of thought, and in return they undo them and give us something fresh. Like when Helena calls Mickey Mouse, Sticky Mouse, or a seagull, a seagoose, and her version is so much better than the rest of the world's.

When it's quiet again, and the beams of headlights skim the concrete, our jackets, the hoods of our cheeks, we bend home, and I come back to that poem.

As a teenager I would take books of poetry to bed, five of my mom's old college books with her name so tidily cursived in the covers, and climb under the blankets even though it was only seven-thirty. It felt like a familiar secret, like I was folding and unfolding some note to myself with these pages so thin and smooth and brown-edged and smelling like only old books can smell. Maybe it was a secret because I never told anyone; maybe it was a secret because I should have been doing something so much more teenagery (at least puffing on a clove if I was going to read poetry). Or maybe it wasn't a secret at all, but just felt like one because it was exciting and comforting at the same time. But I'd read. I always stayed away from the poems that were too long; I just didn't have the patience for them. And some I instantly liked for their simple rhythm, their tragedy or just for the way the words sounded.

But that Emily Dickinson poem? I never liked it. I felt like I should; it was about hope after all, a message of inspiration, a rallying cry for the enduring nature of optimism in the human soul! And yet it wasn't. Something in it was sad. Was it the feathers? Was Dickinson belying hope's permanence with the frailty of that moment before flight? Could the bird just decide to up and go?

Or was it the words? The deadweight of the last line in the first stanza, the deadweight of the word "all" that's far too close to the word fall to leave one with the upturned gaze that hope should supposedly inspire. I mean I'd read it and reread it and I'd always feel ripped off.

But I have it again. Hope. I have hope. However, instead of it making me giddy, making me fling my arms and dance like a thirteen-year-old, instead of it inspiring me to co-opt baby names from national monuments or frozen seafood, I'm just numb.

I don't want hope. I don't want it because it hurts too much when it impales itself on the reality of no. I don't want it for what it never brings. But it's here. The stupid hope is here. Ms. Dickinson is right; it doesn't stop. And maybe her "at all" is only to make it part rhyme with "soul." Or maybe she would have picked that word anyway for the duality and weight it gives to unsolicited optimism.

We get home and Chad fumbles for the key.

"We need to get you in bed, kiddo," I say and lift Helena up. She is so long. Has she grown without me knowing?

And she has weight. Her arms, her long legs, her strong back and little neck, all the weight of rock and bones and stuff that's real, that's really here. I squeeze. Have I missed things while I have been so focused on what isn't here? What have I missed?

"Mama," she says and puts her head on my shoulder.

I put my nose in her hair. Her scalp is warm. My arm fits around her back perfectly. She is from my body. She is her own perfect little body going on in the world.

I look up. Chad is standing on our darkened stoop, both hands holding the keys. Even though his face is in shadow, I think we are looking at each other. I think we are smiling.

I can have this. This husband. This daughter. This house. My hand goes to my belly. And maybe I can have this, too.

17

lood.

"Mama, you should wear a dress today," Helena says as she walks into the bathroom.

"I don't feel like a dress today."

This day will not stop. There is no ref to blow a whistle. I can't go sit on the bench. I have to put clothes on. I have to brush Helena's hair, help her tie her shoes, take keys and put them in the ignition. I have to drop the e-brake and put the car in reverse. I have to drive Helena to school.

"This one has butterflies like my favorite," Helena says and pulls a dress from my messy stack of clothes and puts it on the counter.

I dig for tampons under the sink and only have pads. Definitely a day for yoga pants. Or Harry Potter's invisibility cloak.

Helena leaves the bathroom and returns with more

clothes in her hands. "A dress and jeans and a long sleeve underneath," she says and stacks each item.

Where did you come from? You with your little shoulders back and your eyebrows that go up when you drink. You with your questions about acorns. "Mama, who's this guy?" you asked me yesterday and we crouched in the driveway and talked about trees. You with your jokes and your laugh and the cool side of your face when I kiss you and the smell in your hair that tells me it's you. Where did you come from? And how did you come so easily?

She comes back to the bathroom with a pair of brown high heels. "And these," she says and is already trying to pick up my foot.

"I haven't worn those since before you were born."

"Wear them today. With your dress. And your jeans. And your long sleeve underneath."

"For you, kiddo," I tell her. I kneel down and give her a hug.

"Too tight, Mama," she says.

I know.

I pull on the pants and the long sleeve and the dress. I step into the shoes that make me feel like someone else.

Hours later I'm on my way to pick Helena up from school and my phone rings. I check the caller ID. It's Tracy. I pull over.

"How's it going?"

"Blood," I say. My throat goes tight. My eyes sting. I can't talk through the thick chuffing of breath.

"I'm so sorry," Tracy says.

"I really thought we did it this time," I squeak. I take a breath. "I pinged smiley; we boned like crazy; I had sore boobs and queasiness, but it was PMS all along. I just feel so dumb."

"What's up with pregnancy signs being the same as PMS?" Tracy says. "It's total bullshit."

"I think I'm ready to go to a doctor."

"It might be good. Just see what they say."

"And if they say Clomid? It just seems so unnatural."

"I don't know who you've been talking to," Tracy says, "but the majority of women I know are getting some kind of help. Getting help is natural."

When Chad and I were in graduate school, one of our neighbors was also in school. He was pursuing a PhD in math, a kind of geometry that he'd try to explain by drawing doughnuts in the air and looping his fingers together. He was an artsy mathematician with baggy clothes and a satchel he slung across his chest, who lived in a trailer full of dark paintings and colored candles dripping over the sides of wine bottles. Sometimes he would walk down to our spot and we'd all sit out on our patio and drink and smoke and talk about big things (life, the universe, God, religion, depression, fucked-up relationships) in ways that felt like we were getting somewhere, chipping into the darkness. The alcohol and cigarettes helped us feel smart, and so did having Chris along, with his hands tumbling at his insights and constantly pushing at his hair.

One evening Chris proposed that maybe buildings

and streets and nuclear bombs are just as natural as trees, that anything manmade is still within the dataset of earth and therefore derived from all the same stuff. "Humans can't be outside of nature," he said, "so how can we make anything outside of nature?"

I exhaled and watched the smoke rise and tuned my ears to the constant thrum of the interstate one block over, to the sinusoidal buzz of a semi running east.

"So all of this is meant to be," I said.

"Could be," Chris said, and his cigarette bobbed in his lips.

If I had cancer, I would go to a doctor and take medicine without a second thought. I dye my hair and drink organic milk. I put plug covers on our outlets, wear a seatbelt, lock our doors. I exercise when I don't feel like it, use SPF 50 even though people say it's the same as 15, and call our cats in at night because I worry about raccoons. I spend my life trying to manipulate outcomes, trying to sway odds in my favor and get life to comply with what I want.

So maybe there's nothing different about this. Doing whatever it takes to prevent death should feel just as natural as using science to create life.

That night as we lie in bed, I tell Chad I'm done.

"I can't take this anymore. I'm done with all this. I feel like I'm going crazy."

"With what? All what?" he asks and shifts on his pillow. He is listening now. Frustrated? Scared? Mad? Relieved?

I can't tell, can't read him and this new chalk in his voice. He's waiting.

The room feels too dark even though the walls are mottled with streetlight and shadows and the black edges of definite things. It makes me dizzy. All of it.

"The wondering, all the wondering. The kits, the peeing every morning. Not ovulating. Then ovulating and hoping but telling myself not to hope. The noise. The constant chatter. I want my money back from the damn psychic. I hate him and his February. I want certainty. I want science."

I can tell by the quiet that follows, my last words are being catalogued, tagged and noted, and stored in a tight place. We say so many things that don't matter, but these do.

Science. I have gone to the other side.

18

*h*ave you ever noticed that when you get the things you want, you don't ask questions? I have never been offered a job and wondered why, was never asked out on a date and wondered what it meant. I have never won two bucks on a scratcher lottery ticket and questioned my desire to play the game in the first place. When things go the way I want, the way I expect, it is a tacit confirmation of truths I already carry: I am good enough for the job, I am somebody's good catch, good shit is supposed to happen once in a while. I have an assumption of goodness inside, an innate sense that life is, in fact, good.

But then there are the other times. The times when desires and expectations are left hanging, flapping like empty pillow cases in a laundry-line wind. I don't get the job; I don't even get an interview; my story is rejected for the twenty-seventh time; I see my cat lying on her side beneath the deck and something about the stillness of her small body, the way her paw extends into the dry grass, tells me she is dead.

And these aren't even the doozies. These aren't the stories I hear and read about, the horrific losses humans endure every day—kids dying, homes swept away by hurricanes—but they are still enough to pitch me into the unknown. No matter how often it happens, coming up snake-eyes still feels like being launched into the dark, naked and white fists curling: Why? Why me? What does this mean? What am I supposed to learn?

It's never, for me that I walk away thinking, "Well, that's just how it goes sometimes." And as much as I agree with the bumper sticker "shit happens," when it happens to me, it doesn't feel like it should be happening.

Shit happens to other people, I used to tell myself, lessons happen to me. Because not only has my history shown that good things can come from what seems to be bad, but until now, my survival as a human has depended on believing this. I must find a lesson and make a truth to hold onto. I must make sense of what has thrown me into chaos.

"Maybe this is God's way of telling you something," my Christian friend Noel told me when I confided in her about not being able to get pregnant. I love Noel, but I didn't love the way her tight smile apparently knew what the Big Cheese was up to.

"Yeah," I said, hoping she would stop. Despite our differences in belief, we had always been able to get beyond semantics and hear each other from a place of love. But that day, I wasn't in the mood.

"Maybe it's His way of saying you should just relax," Noel continued, "that you are not in control."

"Like your situation," I said cutting her off. If we got talking about her life, maybe she wouldn't say what I was afraid she was thinking. I wanted to stop her before she got on a roll, before she used my moment of vulnerability to make the case for Jesus or suggest that not being able to have a kid was somehow linked to my not being Christian. All I needed was for her to make one of those geometric proofs, a simple if/then statement, when, in fact, nothing about any of this is clean.

As much as I, too, need to tell myself something, I also know we are all just humans reaching, groping for something outside of ourselves to mollify our pain. Use religion, use reason, use Shakespeare or Jung. Use your dreams, your fortune cookies, the way the birds take flight in the sky. Use your horoscope, the wisdom of your grandmother, the homeless guy on the Tijuana bridge who hunched over his hand and said, "You haven't found him yet." Signs, all signs from what we want to know is there: certainty. Someone, please tell us there are certain things.

And we don't need certainty when we don't have doubt.

When I was in graduate school, I stood slanted in the hall waiting for a professor. He approached in that fast-stepped way professors walk and said, "Reading *Moby Dick*?" and started unlocking his office with the jingle of keys. "What do you think?"

I looked at the copy wedged in my arm, the same copy I had to buy in high school and had never read even though my wild-eyed English teacher whom I adored said it was his favorite book. "I love it," I said. I was reading it this time, and was loving it; who could read the first page without feeling instant kinship with the November in Ishmael's soul?

"Have you gotten to the doubloon chapter yet?"

"No."

"It's my favorite chapter," he said and leaned back in his chair with his chin up and a wicked grin bending his mustache straight.

"It's good, huh?" I asked and glowed.

"It's good," he said. "Wait till you get there."

I asked him my credits question, and as I was leaving his office, he said, "The doubloon chapter. I think you'll like it."

As if I could forget.

So Ahab in his mad quest to kill Moby Dick nails a doubloon to the mast of the Pequod as a reward for whichever man spots the white whale. And as it hangs, many men approach and reflect on what they see. And although the coin does not change, is not even flipped on its other side, each man looks into its gold surface stamped with mountains and a sun and sees something different.

Ahab sees himself. Starbuck sees the Trinity. Stubb sees the human experience. Flask sees what he can buy.

What has always struck me about this chapter is how well it illustrates our search for truth, the way we all can read the same signs and interpret them differently. And in a way, since reading this chapter, it has become a truth of its own: We all must interpret; we all must think our truth is true.

Until now this has been enough. It has felt like a realization, something that cuts through the bullshit and hypocrisy of so much dogma. But it doesn't go beyond that, it doesn't cover what's left after I stand around in a crowd of humans and observe, judge even. What then? Where do I go with my own doubt and cynicism and wonder? I know what I'm not, but what am I?

I am jealous for one. I am jealous of the person before the mast locked in one way of thinking. How peaceful it must be to be united in spirit and belief to the disregard of any other possibility.

But I can't be that.

So I will be none of it. I will step out of the ring of truth-making and into the objective side of certainty. Science, with its cells and molecules and machines. I will get knowledge and answers and resolutions. I will fix whatever is wrong.

Despite months of "letting whatever happen" to months of ovulation predictor kits to months of charting and having sex perfectly timed, I am still not pregnant after what is now almost three years of hoping. Something is obviously wrong. All this "if it's meant to be, it will happen" mumbo-jumbo could be compromised by the simple fact of scar tissue in a fallopian tube, low sperm count, or like Tracy discovered after going to a fertility specialist, a four-inch cyst on an ovary.

Then what about the miscarriage from a year ago?

There may not have been a heartbeat, but I did get pregnant.

Maybe something has changed. Maybe my deepest deeps are riddled with tangible problems that can be detected, diagnosed and ultimately set right.

Fix me, Doc. Just fix me.

19

*d*r. Platt is a short, lashless man who wears pleated pants and has the same stay-in-place-good-boy haircut he surely had on graduation day, circa 1985. He smiles and shakes my hand and as we walk down the hall I feel like I'm following a preppy Ewok on the way to the ninth hole. But I figure if he has the keys, keys to anything (my ovaries, the little stubborn drying up eggs, or the key to any kind of certainty, even if it's "I'm sorry, you just can't have kids") then I shouldn't make *Star Wars* comparisons unless it's going to be to Han Solo.

Dr. Platt takes a seat behind a desk that is so big he's looking more like R2-D2 perched in the X-wing fighter. He starts flipping through my chart in the same way you flip through a book when you tell a friend, "Let me just read you this one part." Except he doesn't have a smirk of excitement. He's just flipping.

"So you have been able to get pregnant. You've just

been having difficulty."

"Yes," I say and exhale. He's going to look up any minute, going to give me my big cue to unload the goods. At least he has to give me that smidge of doctor eye contact, that feigned warm-eyed glimpse that starts the thirty seconds you have before your throat is fondled and rubber gloves are being snapped off and tossed in the trash.

But Dr. Platt keeps his head down. Keeps flipping. "So the D and C was a year ago?"

"Yes," I say. At least he knows about the miscarriage. Knows I have been through that.

Back to flipping. He has a pleasant look on his face. He might even be smiling.

"It's good to see you smiling," I say. He doesn't look up. Does he know what I'm trying to do? "I mean it's good to see someone smiling in all of this."

Come on, Doc, toss me a bone. Say something so we can connect. Look up and give me an indication that you know what Chad and I have been through. Maybe say, "I know it can be tough" or "What have you all done so far?" or hey, if you want to send me to the moon, maybe actually say, "Tell me about it." Can you imagine if he said, "Tell me about it" and meant it?

Dr. Platt looks up, but not far enough to see the flash of his eyes, just the slope of his nose. He looks back down so he's all hair again. "Well you're here and now it's my job to get you pregnant."

I think there's a joke I could crack here, and if I were in another mood I might risk it, but I'm shaky and starting to dislike the little dude on the other side of the desk.

Forget about even being on the side of the Force; Dr. Platt is starting to look like one of those Gamorrean pig guards in Jabba's palace. I keep my trap shut and wonder why I'm not relieved. What he said is what I want to hear right? Getting me pregnant is what we're here to do. So why does his confidence and the simplicity of his statement feel empty? Why do I still feel cold and alone?

Dr. Platt rolls to a file cabinet and pulls out a glossy piece of paper. He sets it between us.

"This gives you an overview of the process," he says, and taps his pen on a corner of the sheet. I glance down and see names with x's and v's and purple angled swoops and thickly lettered font. I see pharmaceutical companies. How much money do they pay some ad team to come up with the presentation of these drugs? The names alone are surely Kama Sutra-ing my subconscious into various contortions as I sit here dumb. Dr. Platt keeps talking. "Typically we do some testing and we wait for your period so that on your next cycle we can get you on a round of drugs."

"Actually, my last gynecologist suggested drugs about a year-and-a-half ago."

"Did you try them?" Dr. Platt asks. For the first time he is actually looking up with his whole face.

"No. My husband and I both have some issues with using the drugs. We are more focused on the diagnostic angle to see if anything is wrong."

"We can test, we can test," he says. "But usually the tests come back fine, and I write you a prescription and get the process started. At your age you have a two to five percent chance of getting pregnant on your own. It's just the way it is. So most people opt for the drugs as a starting point."

"What about multiples?"

"There is a one-in-ten chance of multiples, and even then it's usually just twins."

Just twins. Can you come over at two in the morning when my twins are screaming? Can I get you to kick-in for the third college fund? Can I call you when this third child is heartbroken or stoned or depressed or hunched over in teenage angst asking me why he was ever born? And what do I tell him—"Actually it's your sister we wanted, you were just part of the two-for-one special"? How can someone ever say "just" when referring to someone's life and all of its unforeseen complexity? And how can he say "just" to the parents who bear responsibility for that life?

Should I even be here?

If this had been four-and-a-half years ago and we had never been able to get pregnant, I think I would feel completely different. If Clomid were the only way I thought I could get pregnant, I would have figured that it was meant to be and I would have stepped into the process and accepted the odds of twins. But I don't think it's the only way to get pregnant because I've already gotten pregnant. My shit works, or has worked, so what is wrong with it now?

"Even twins is a lot for us," I say.

"Well, when we scan the follicles, if more than one is maturing, you can abstain from having sex if you're that worried about it. But truthfully, with someone like you, we'd probably want more than one egg, maybe two to four, to come out to increase the chances."

Someone like you? What's that supposed to mean? Someone with brown hair? Two cats? Overly obsessed with becoming pregnant? He means something, but it's obviously not what Rod Stewart meant.

"Can we just start with the testing and see where we go from there?"

When I get home I call Chad.

"What's wrong?" he asks.

"Nothing's wrong. It was fine."

"But what is it? Why do you sound like that?"

"What?"

"Disappointed," he says.

So I tell him. I tell him how quickly Dr. Platt read my chart. How he never asked what we had been through or how we were doing. How he never asked what we wanted. How he balked at my questions and referred me to a worksheet. How there was a process, a checklist to go through. How his answers always ended with one thing: drugs.

"Can I say something?" Chad says.

"What?"

"We lay in bed and you said you wanted certainty. You said you wanted science. He's not there to make you feel good. He's there to give you results. This is what science is."

He's right. And science is what I want. Sperms and eggs and numbers. And if nothing else, just start with the tests.

So I peed and gave blood. Chad jacked off in a cup. Dr. Platt squirted dye into my uterus and fallopian tubes while I arched my back to look at the screen.

Two weeks later I am sitting in Dr. Platt's office again.

"Tracy?" Dr. Platt says and smiles and holds out his hand to shake. He's looking me in the eyes. Ahhh, yes, today I'm getting the kinder, gentler Dr. Platt. The Dr. Platt 2.0. He takes a seat behind his battle station. "We got all of your results. Normal. Everything looks great. And your husband's numbers look really good."

Oh, yippee harahoe, we're all normal! Time to crack open the bubbly!

Normal? Normal means there's nothing wrong. Normal means there's nothing to fix. Why can't there be something to fix?

Dr. Platt grins and takes out a prescription pad. "You can get this at any pharmacy."

"But what about PCOS or UFS? You never did an ovary ultrasound. Should we test for that first?" I had checked my fertility bible, boned up on whatever could be wrong.

"UFS is something that a lot of people don't even believe in. It can happen, but it's not proven. And with PCOS you have to have two out of three of these symptoms: irregular periods, long periods, cycles without ovulation."

"But I have all of those," I say.

"Look, you can do whatever you want." His hands come up as he leans back in his chair, and I realize I have seen him before; I have taught a few kids like him. He's that B plus student who does most of his work and answers questions when asked but never volunteers anything. He's the kind of kid who smiles when he's looking at you but stares mean into the face of his desk when you're looking away. He's the kid who quietly takes his hat off when you ask except for on a random Tuesday when he says, "I said I'd do it!" even though you hadn't asked a second time.

"If I do go with the drugs, is it true there's only a thirty percent success rate?"

"Thirty percent? It's probably more like fifteen percent for a person your age." I do some quick subtraction (yes, Dr. Platt, despite my senility, I can still borrow a one!) and remind myself that I'm thirty-seven and not eighty-six. "Look," he says and leans in, "your uterus is like a black box. I can only do so much. We can up your eggs and insert sperm. We can even do IVF. But I can't control what goes on inside that box. I can't give you any guarantees."

"You can't give me certainty?"

"No. Not at all."

I tell Chad the results of all the tests and how there are no problems. I tell him about the drug conversation and I find myself leaving out my aversion to it. I say, "I asked about the thirty percent success rate and the doctor said really it's only fifteen percent." But instead of saying it in a way that evokes the subtext of "Can you believe that even on the drugs there is still only fifteen percent chance of success?" I am saying it bleakly as if to say, "Even with Clomid there is a small chance of success. So Clomid is kind of a mystery, too. It's not a guaranteed presto-change-o." Does this mean I want to do it? Why am I trying to make it sound good to him?

Chad just listens, and when I finish, I am quiet, too. A year ago I would press him right now, ask him what he's thinking, demand some kind of response. But focusing on his decision would just be a way to avoid focusing on mine.

I'm not sure when we will talk about it, but I know we will.

I can't stop all the thoughts from swarming like a ball of eels. Getting pregnant is a biological process. It's sperm and egg uniting. It's being in the right place in the right time. Why not try the drugs? Why not up the odds? It's no different than doing ovulation predictor kits, really. It's not like they are eggs from a hybrid chicken-goat, or eggs manufactured in a plant whose commercials I can just imagine: "Humenz" (insert woman running in field, ala the maxi pad ads, running in white pants and hopping like a fleecy lamb) "eggs for the eggless!" That's not even me. The eggs are already there. The drugs would just help them out.

But there's something else I keep thinking about, too. Months and months ago, before we moved, Noel asked me to go with her to hear a Christian inspirational speaker. I went, and it's something this guy said that keeps looping in my head. He was talking about prayers, about how you should pray and how you shouldn't be afraid to ask for anything. "But people always think that when their prayer doesn't come true, that God isn't answering it, that he's not listening," the man had said, leaning into the crowd, "but God is always listening. It's just that sometimes His answer is no." I had laughed the way I had laughed the first time I heard Eddie Murphy impersonate a white person. My god, it's true! We are like that! I never assume the answer is no. I never think no is meant to be. But maybe it is. And maybe it's not even no in that solid clarified way of someone just telling me, "No, it can't happen." Instead it's no in the unsatisfying way of a prayer seeped from my heart cracked open and floating dimly around the moth-filled light. It's a constant prayer whose no is found in the equal match of constant silence.

Later that day I call Mom. I tell her our tests are normal. I tell her the doctor keeps suggesting the drugs.

As usual I'm in two places at once. "I just don't want to wait and decide to do the drugs three months from now," I tell her. "If Clomid is going to feel right three months from now, I'd just rather start it now."

"I guess I'd be asking myself if there was any way at all we'd consider the drugs. If the answer is yes, then it does seem like you should start them now. But if it's no, it's no." She pauses. "What is your gut telling you?" she says.

My gut? Do I even have a gut anymore?

But I do. And I know I do. It's not the noisy brain banter of Sophie and Merle, but it's that other voice, the quiet one who has been there all along. But I don't like it. I don't like what it knows.

"Doing the Clomid just doesn't feel right. It just doesn't." I sigh. It feels sad. It feels scary. But it's the truth. It's the quiet blue line of truth.

That night Chad and I decide to talk. He tells me he doesn't want to do the Clomid. I tell him I don't either. I am so glad to be sitting with him in agreement. And I'm relieved to have made a decision. Even though we've decided on continued ambiguity, it just feels good to scratch something off the list.

"I'll just keep doing the ovulation predictors and that's it."

"Sounds good," he says and stretches his arms up then puts each hand on the edge of the chair.

"It was good meeting with you, Chad," I say.

"Thanks, Tracy," he raises and lowers his eyebrows. He puts his hand on his chin and looks up, then flips his finger out to point. "I'll have my secretary type up the minutes and get those to you by noon tomorrow."

"But seriously," I say and look at my hands.

"Seriously," Chad says in his regular voice. But I can't feel him, can't feel all of him. But I want to.

"I think I'll go to bed early," I say.

"I guess I will, too," he says and grins.

20

We made love. Normal, beautiful, unplanned love.

The next morning I pee on a stick while Chad stands at the sink in his work shirt and brushes his teeth.

☺

"Hey, check that out," I say and show him. I had thought maybe I wouldn't be fertile this month, but here it is. The eyes! The smile! And we even had sex last night! Maybe the psychic was just off by a month. Because something about this time is definitely different. We had unplanned sex the night before the smiley face just like we did with Helena; I am using the sticks in front of Chad so there aren't any more secrets; and I kind of sort of have opened myself up to the possibility that it may not happen at all. Okay, okay, I am silently chuckling to the universe, joke's on us. This is when it's meant to happen. "So you think we can do it tonight and the next night?" I ask Chad.

"Of course," Chad says without a pause. I looked at his reflection. He doesn't look at me, but spits and rinses and heads downstairs to eat. Does he really mean "of course"? There was some faint echo of a borrowed phrase in there, some automatic response he's preprogrammed into his repertoire. He's going through something, has been going through some journey of his own that we don't talk about, something that would make him develop this kind of response. Just do it, I can imagine him telling himself, no matter how you feel or what resentments you have, when she comes to you with the question, you better give her the green light.

Maybe I'll ask him someday. But not now. Not now when we just need two more days of seed.

That night is fine. Nice even. But the next day Chad gets busy building a pantry for our kitchen. It's a Saturday and I beg him to go to a birthday party for one of Helena's classmates. I don't want to go alone.

"Can't you guys go without me so I can get some work done?" Chad asks. "When else can I do this stuff? I only have the weekends."

"Please?"

He goes. We watch Helena make a pizza and sit at a long table with other kids. When we get home he returns to the tape measurer, the saw and the boards.

We have been here before, the time when my dad and stepmom were visiting. Even though this time he's not wearing eye, ear, and hand protection, I feel threatened by his focus, his ability to get lost in projects. Does he remember that tonight is the third night? The one he preapproved thirty-six hours ago? Everything about this time has been going so well; can't we just finish it off?

When Chad breaks for dinner and is slumped in front of a frozen pizza, I say, "How about a quickie and then I'll stay up and watch a movie while you work on the pantry?"

He looks to the empty space in front of him. He turns to me, "Do we have to?"

No.

No, we don't.

It's new, a new and calm voice. It's wise and peaceful, and straight out of nowhere but in me, somewhere inside me. And I know this is one of those times. So often I mistake the external crossroads I face every few years (go to Ecuador/not go to Ecuador, take the job/not take the job) as the really important ones when actually the important ones are these: the gazillion internal crossroads faced each day, hundreds of thoughts and responses and reactions, hundreds of chances to do things from a new place, some new and different place. These are the crossroads of practice, the frayed paths of pattern-breaking that eventually change us into the person we're trying to be. And here is one of those opportunities. Just like the tagged and runned base that's too close to call when B and I'd play Wiffle Ball in the street—this is the do-over. No, we don't have to.

"Yes," I say. My hands come to my hips. "We have to."

"Okay," Chad says. He looks away.

My hands drop and reach for the dishtowel and fold it over the oven handle. I pull it until both sides hang even.

What kind of compromise can there be? Tell him we don't have to, then be swamped with regret thirteen days later when I get my period? What about the couple in the fertility book, the man with the back injury who was tired and in pain and his wife rode him like a jockey and that was the night their son was conceived? It just takes one time. One time!

One time, I want to yell at Chad. The existence of our future kid could be hanging on this one time!

Fuck the do-over.

I go upstairs.

We are in our bedroom. It is dark, but light from our closet makes some things seen. Chad grabs for his pants and pushes his legs inside. His belt rattles. Change in his pocket jingles. His feet are loud on the wood floor as he leaves. He's on the stairs, but I can hear him. He says, "No, I'm not walking away. We are going to finish this." His slippered feet thump and get louder.

I am on the bed, sitting. My t-shirt is on, but my underwear is still in a knot on top of my folded pajama bottoms in a stack on the floor. I had put them there next to the bed so the plan would be completely smooth. Sex: check. Jammies without having to stand: check. Linger in the bed doing pelvis tilt for thirty minutes: check. Go downstairs to watch movie all glowy-glowy and complete while Chad bangs some nails: check. March attempt successful: check! Check! Check!

But it hadn't gone that way at all.

Chad closes the bedroom door. "I won't get mad, but

I just need to vent. Why did you stop?" he asks. "You stopped things, right? Because I could have kept going. I don't want to take the blame here."

"Yeah," I say. "I did stop. I just couldn't."

We had been in the middle of the quickie, the one I said we absolutely must have before returning to our evening, and I had stopped things. His kisses had felt so empty and foreign. It hadn't even been a choice or a thought; my body had just recoiled.

"I don't think I can do this much longer," Chad says and his hands go to his hair and drop to the space in front of his chest. "This issue has been the toughest challenge in our marriage. For me. Watching you go through this every time. I can't deal."

In the past, when I gave him the okay to vent, I would listen, but I'd be focusing on something else, scanning his words for a way out, listening for some kind of transgression so I could be right about something and sway the power dynamic in my favor. I'd be listening for all the ways he was wrong and listening for all the points I could rebut. But the rebuttals aren't coming. Chad is talking. His mouth is moving and his hands are moving heavy like he is wearing weighted gloves.

"It's been building for a while," he says. "I haven't talked to anyone, and I've just been trying to ignore it, but I can't anymore."

I used to ask Chad to tell me stories. We'd be walking or driving or sitting around on a hot day and I'd ask him to tell me about Billy. Billy had been a friend of Chad's who had lived across the street when Chad was a kid. Billy had seven siblings whose names all started with the letter B. Billy loved trains and got crappy mustard sandwiches in his lunch. He had a mom who yelled and a one-armed dad who tried to start his car on a cold morning but flooded the engine and beat the dash with his good arm until the car shook and his stump jerked. Billy had headaches and drew forts. But when Chad wanted to build them, Billy would complain about his head and go inside.

Even though I knew how the stories would end, I wanted to hear more. I loved Billy. I loved Chad as a kid loving Billy with his top button always buttoned. And I started to wonder if that's what love was: the telling and the keeping of each other's stories as if they were our own.

It has been so long since I have asked Chad to tell me a story.

"It was for you. I did this for you." Chad stops. He looks at me. He pulls at the front of his hair. "I used to be happy with what we have. I used to think the three of us was a beautiful thing. And I don't anymore. With you and your disappointment and your feeling that something is missing. You with your ups and downs. It's nuts. I have it and I don't want it. I want what I used to have. Us. The three of us. And you can't give it back," Chad says. He wipes his eyes. "You're the one who took it. But you can't give it back."

I'm faint and frilly, like looking over the edge of a bridge or to the tiny ground from the top of a building. What have I done? What have I done?

"This whole thing is so divisive to our relationship. It's not worth it."

Here it comes.

"I just don't think I want to keep trying. I don't want to keep trying. I can't do it," Chad says and straightens. "I'm done."

I run my nails along the tick-tick of stitches of the quilt on our bed to feel something like earth. I try to smile.

"But if you could," Chad says, "you would just keep going through this in the same way until you get pregnant. Every month, the same. And the whole time we're here; Helena and I are right here in front of you. We're here now."

"Thanks for saying all of this."

"And you don't even see it."

"I'm not mad," I hear my voice from the outside, "but can we stop talking?"

I get up and go to the bathroom. I leave the light off and sit on the lid of the toilet. I breathe. Breathe. I can see her, the little girl, my other daughter. Her hair is curly and dark and she has a space between her front teeth. She is standing on the beach in her little swimsuit with the surf loud behind her, and she is smiling big like someone has asked her to smile for a picture and she is making the joke on them. She smiles so big her eyes close. She opens them. She opens them and waves.

When people would ask Chad and me how we met, I would always get excited. I loved that ours was a story, a real story with extraordinary events and fraught with so many ways it might not have been.

"You tell it," I would say to Chad. I wanted to hear it

from his mouth, wanted to hear him, so I would know he believed in the magic of us.

"No, you tell," he'd say.

"So I was half way down my stairs when I decided to go back inside and change my sweater," I would start.

"Prepare yourself," Chad would say rolling his eyes to the listener. "She's going for the long version."

I would continue anyway, suspecting that he was dissenting for the amusement value. But I would look at him, too, while I was talking, and he'd be listening with his head to the side and his arm swung around the back of a chair as if he were just another dinner guest, not one of the lead stars.

"You don't like it when I tell our story," I said once, whispering in the dark of our hosts' loft.

"I do like it."

"When I look at you, you seem annoyed or something."

"No, I'm not annoyed," he said.

"Why don't you ever want to tell it?"

"You tell it better. I like listening to you tell it."

"Really, you're not annoyed?"

"No."

It wasn't until last month during one of those traffic light reflections, when one hand was on the steering wheel and the other was in my lap or on the e-brake or drumming on some part of the dash, that I realized that our story has never really been ours; it has only ever been mine. Chad wasn't there when I decided to change my shirt, or park my car, or when I heard some bearded stranger yelling at me to get out of the way. He hadn't felt thankful to be alive and had a mechanic turn him away such that he ended up at Rino's Shell. He had just been at work, like any other day, wiping his greasy hands on a rag when some woman walked in to use the phone. He had decided to talk to her and ask her about the college on her sweatshirt in the same way nineteen thousand other men and women strike up conversations with each other.

I wasn't sure at the time why the thought had occurred then, out of nowhere, but as the light went green and I eased through the intersection I said out loud, "Trip out on that." Trip out that it has taken me eight years to realize his side of things. In eight years I had never really realized that he had never been there to experience all the magic I had; he had only heard me talk about it and constantly sling it about like a weekend suitcase I was happily obliged to bring.

As I sit in the dark picturing this little girl, the girl who has been fated to come, I am thankful for that traffic-stop thought and how it prepared me for this. The desire to have a second child, the creation of her image, her little laugh, her tenacity and irreverence, are all my doing. Chad has never wanted any of it in the same way. He hasn't felt it in the same way. He is definitely not saying goodbye to something that, to him, has never existed.

I wave back to her. I kneel in the sand and hug her and feel her black curls fluff on my arm. I made you. I made you, and I will keep you close. I don't need to wait for meant to be.

You are already here.

21

i keep having imaginary conversations with Tracy or my mom.

"I think we're finally giving up."

"We've decided to stop trying."

"We're going to drop the whole thing."

I'm not sure which sounds better, but they all sound okay, like pieces of river rock chucked back to the bed.

So I look online for jobs. I write a friend in Ecuador and wonder when we can see him. I think about cute clothes I can buy if I am working and we have more money. I can come back to myself, and Chad and I can get back to our old relationship wherein conversations go uninterrupted for hours and matinees can be seen in the middle of the afternoon. We can scuba dive again.

"Remember the trailer?" Chad says one night in bed. It's dark, but I know we're both looking at the ceiling.

"Good times," I say, parroting some visor-wearing

neighbor we had met who had asked us if we were from "Cali."

"Remember David," Chad says talking about the man who had lived next to us, "sitting on his tailgate with his music going all night?"

"¿Quieres una fria?" I impersonate Dave.

"It was small, but we had that place dialed."

"We had to. Except for the couch. My half was always a sty."

"We lived in that trailer four years," Chad says.

"And the railroad tracks were right there," I say. "And the whole trailer would shake."

"Remember how you'd always want to cross the tracks to check mail?"

"I just liked checking mail."

"I know but every night."

"Well, you know," I say. "Those were the days."

"When you just never knew? When something great was going to happen?"

"Yeah."

"They're gone?"

"I think so."

"No," Chad says and makes the word long. He slides a hand over my hip. "That's sad."

"It's not, though," I say. "I think great things are here. I just haven't been seeing them."

A few days later Chad and I push Helena in her stroller and walk downtown. It's a bright day with high wind and nothing but blue sky. People are out, as if we all got the same memo. A man and woman are walking in front of us, his arm draped around her shoulders. They stop and kiss and laugh and continue to walk in that slow, hip-swaying way of having no place to go.

"Second marriage?" I say to Chad.

"Probably."

"Kids?"

"None from each other. Or if so they have long since left the house."

"Maybe it's still new," I say. "You know, they get to do it all over again. Have a life with kids, get divorced, then start all over again with someone else when the kids are gone. It's a whole new life. Looks like it could be kind of fun." Chad looks at me. "Instead of, you know," I say heavily, "the daily grind we are in." He laughs.

But I want some of that back. I want to be dawdling in the slow-grin world on a Sunday afternoon with Chad. I want to feel the ease of our silly importance like we used to.

So giving up on having another child is right for all of us: for me, for Chad, for our relationship. It is in our best interests as a family, financially, emotionally, and spiritually.

That's what I've been telling myself all week. And sometimes when I'm walking or driving and I have the thought, you could be pregnant; you still haven't gotten your period and you guys did have sex on key days, I shut it out. I see the dark curly-haired girl running. I tell myself to look away. She only exists in your head.

By the end of the week, I am in the car waiting to turn,

my blinker ticking softly.

You could be pregnant.

Oh no.

Did you just say oh no? Did you really mean it? Or have you just been brainwashing yourself?

I take a deep breath.

I mean it. I don't want to be pregnant.

Check that out—the light turns green; I let my foot off the break—I've finally arrived.

But that was before today.

I felt back cramps last night. And I thought I could see a faint pink streak on the toilet paper this morning. My period is coming and with it the reality. The real reality.

I am not pregnant again.

And now, with everything we've decided, I really may never be.

I just feel so quiet.

Just don't cry. Crying will undo everything. Crying will mean that none of it mattered. Crying will mean nothing is new.

I drive Helena to school. I am so lost in my own thoughts that we are halfway there when I remember she is in the car, too. As usual, when I think of her, she knows. She snaps from her own quietude in song, "I'll meet you at the top of the coconut tree." This is the kind of one-liner from silence that usually gets me to turn around even though I'm driving, to sling one arm behind the seat and to grab her knee or poke her side until she giggles and knows that I know she has just cracked a joke. It's one of the ways we are to each other: a series of half-thoughts, jumbled words, mixed lines from songs, a way we cast a feeler to the other to say hello or I love you or I know you out of everyone in the universe.

But I can't answer her because if I open my mouth my heart will flop out, raw and wet and still beating.

"Mama, do you remember that one?" Helena asks.

Take a deep breath. Swallow. "I do."

She continues with the rhyme, her words so rounded and full and completely not the right ones from the song.

She's beautiful.

No matter how much not having a second child might be right for me, for Chad, for our marriage, I don't know if I'll ever be convinced it's right for Helena. I in my take-myself-so-seriously adult persona can never give her the kind of silliness a sibling could. She won't have stinky feet in her face on road trips, uncontrollable giggles at the dinner table, mean words slung and forgiven, and the solid certainty through it all that someone shares a piece of who she is in a way that can never be replicated.

"What do I tell her?" I ask Tracy when I call her later that morning. "What do I tell her when she asks me why we never gave her a brother or a sister?"

Tracy does not hesitate. "You tell her because she's enough."

22

*t*he light is off, but I can see something dark on the toilet paper. I flip on the light.

Oh.

And before anything can sink, I tell myself, say it in my head: You'll be okay. You'll be okay.

I step out of the bathroom and Chad is standing there in just his underwear.

"Have you gotten your period?" he says.

"Yes."

"When?"

"Just right now."

His eyes drop.

"But I'm okay."

He still looks down; my words don't give him relief.

I hug him and he slumps on me and I hug him even tighter.

I'm not sure what his sadness means, but I don't think

I will ask. This game has been too complex. To ask and make him stand behind words would only be so I could work it into the equation: So does this mean he does really want a kid? Does this mean he does want to try Clomid? I can't do it anymore. If I truly want to know, the only way I will let myself ask is if I am asking to hear about him, to listen to his experience, as a friend, as someone who's had his journey on his own. I have never really done that, ask him how he is, what he is experiencing without trying to use his response for my final outcome, to feed my own desire. Even though I never would have seen it at the time, I have been so selfish in all of this, so focused, at the expense of who knows what.

"I'm hiding!" Helena calls from our bed. Some time while I was in the bathroom, she must have climbed in, and apparently we've been playing hide-and-seek and kept her waiting for years.

I jump on the bed and squeeze where the tent of the blankets is the highest. I think I have her belly. She laughs. "Then why are you telling us you're hiding?" I say and tickle her more.

She lowers the cover so I can see her wild hairdo puffing around her. She frowns. "No, Mama, we are playing hide-and-seek."

"I thought we were playing hide-and-tell," I say. I kiss her. I kiss her and go downstairs.

When I see it's still early, I decide we can walk to Helena's school instead of driving. I've always wanted to try it, but since her school is miles away, the timing has been tough.

"If you get dressed right now, we can do it," I tell Helena when she finishes her cereal.

"You're nuts," Chad says, and I kind of know he's right, but I also know we are going for it.

Maybe you are just running, trying to run from the reality of your period. Maybe you are just trying to stay in motion because if you stand still you will break down. Maybe you thought you'd be all okay with it, and really that was bullshit, too, and you are on the brink and back where you started only you are just trying to cover it up by pushing a stroller for hours.

Maybe.

I am sitting in front of Helena's dresser now, holding up a pair of pants that she doesn't want to put on. I could not go. I could drive. And I'm glad the thought comes easily. Glad that I can let go of my plan. Things might not go my way.

Helena picks some pants of her own. I get dressed, and we say goodbye to Chad. I step outside and start to walk. The light is still yellow morning light, and the cool has stayed pocketed on our street. This is why I want to walk. It just feels good.

We make it to Helena's school in exactly one hour, and after dropping her off, I turn around and appreciate the lightness of the stroller. It never feels like pushing a stroller should count as resistance training, but the ease with which I'm cruising home and the fact that I'm actually walking upright with my butt in the same zip code as my head, I realize it is.

Half way home my head is still buzzing with thoughts:

See, now you can move on to all the other things you want to do in life; now you can just focus on the three of you; it is okay, your body can truly be your own again.

Wow, look how you are already back at it. Look how you are already picking up the brush and the paints and stepping up to the canvas once more. And I think of Melville again, of *Moby Dick*.

At the end of the book, Ishmael is left the only survivor, left bobbing on a coffin in the middle of the ocean. At the end of the semester, I wrote a paper theorizing that Melville left Ishmael alive because he was the only character who could withstand uncertainty. Everyone else: Queequeg, Pip, Starbuck, Ahab, men who either had unquestioned truth or men who had doubted their truth but had redoubled their rote belief in an effort to erase all doubt, got waxed. It is Ishmael and his observations, his questions, his empty-handedness who is still breathing and sane by the end. It's as if Melville is saying that being human is about uncertainty, so let it be. Or maybe Melville is not saying that, but the book is the doubloon, and that's what I'm saying.

Something will become clear in time, I think, as I pop the front wheel of the stroller onto the curb. Or it may not.

Twenty minutes later I'm almost home. I see a mother across the street walking with an infant in one arm and a three-year-old walking and holding onto her other hand. I look away.

But you'll be able to do other things, travel, scuba dive, get back to the other life.

But what if that's never enough? What if you always

have a hole? What if you lose the fifteen pounds and go get your teeth whitened and go to Italy and have date nights with Chad and wear cute outfits all the time and it still isn't enough?

Then you will find a cause to dedicate yourself to. You and Chad and Helena will do whale research or pollution research or go live for a year in Thailand and help build houses for others. You will do something to help the environment and people and kids.

Then what about adoption? You want a cause, how about truly loving a child who doesn't have a home?

I turn left on my block and realize I have been doing it again: letting the answers come too easily, letting possibilities fuel excitement because excitement is what I want to feel. Maybe that's just how the brain works; when I am in pain, my brain wants to step in and bail me out.

Maybe you just need a good meditation class.

Or maybe just a hit of some crazy-good weed!

So much for Sophie and Merle.

Enter Spicoli.

But there is probably a kid out there who could use a home.

The thought comes in the voice of the dog that's been told not to bark but has to get in that last grumbly half-bark before he's going to be quiet.

Yes, I think to the voice, picture petting its worried head, I hear you. I hear you, but that doesn't mean I have to listen.

☺

When I gave up or gave in, when I succumbed to not having control over getting pregnant, my head was so much quieter. I was left with what was in front of me: grass and the sun in trees, the smell of Helena's hair, Chad bringing home fifty-cent Nutty Bars and two Sprites and decisions about whether to watch *Bourne Identity* or a documentary about how art changed the lives of garbage sorters in Brazil.

I guess you could say, without realizing it, I finally (I hate to say it) relaxed.

And guess what happened?

"Chad," I whispered in predawn darkness.

"What is it?"

"I'm pregnant."

And guess what happened after that?

The doctor said spotting was normal at six weeks and that the heart rate looked good.

"There's a heartbeat?" I asked.

"Yes," she said and she turned it loud enough that the

speaker static hung on the edges of the beat so each pump was knit like a fuzzy sweater to the last: pshh-pshh, pshh-pshh.

"It sounds good," the doctor said. "It looks good."

When I showed Chad the pictures of the ultrasound, he took them and stared. He stood up and grinned and swatted at me like a spanking.

"What?" I said.

"See?" He stretched the word long like he had known something all along, like I had worried for nothing.

That evening the spotting turned to blood. The nurse said there was nothing I could do. Nothing they could do.

The next ultrasound showed a fuzzy screen—no black sac, no slushy beating heart.

"Was it a person?" Chad asked. We were sitting on the bed. His arms hung down and his hands turned up in his lap, his fingers like they'd been ripped from dirt.

"I don't know," I said.

"I just wish I hadn't known about the heart." The fingers rose to his face. Pushed at his eyes.

"I know."

"How many times can people go through this? Heartbeats then no heartbeats?"

"I don't know." Some seconds passed. I scrambled for something to say. But there was no answer, no tidy bow to tie up the mess of hurt. "I just know it's a part of us," I said. "Everything we've been through. The trying, the not trying. The heartbeat. The no heartbeat. All of it."

When I told my mom, she said perspective only comes with time. I knew she was trying to help, trying to give me some kind of hope, but I told her I don't believe in perspective anymore. I told her it's only something the brain offers our heart, only something we try to offer each other when we don't know what to say.

Later, I realized this may have sounded angry or resentful, like something flung from the mouth of someone who feels ripped off. And there is a part of me deep down that does feel ripped off, but that's not why I said it. The bigger part of me, the better part of me, said it because I'm afraid of reaching for things like perspective. Perspective means wanting to feel something other than what I'm feeling right now. Perspective means putting value in the long view and its inevitable truth that will strive to make a mess neat. Perspective means thinking I've got something figured out. I don't want to figure anything out. And if I need to know something, if I do need something solid to lean on in the face of so much uncertainty, I will lean on now. Right now, with its hurt and beautiful grit. Right now, with its minutes that go and go and go and cannot be relived.

All this time that I've been waiting for meant to be, have been busy trying to make meant to be, I've been missing out on what is.

What simply is.

We're at the park. It's a hazy-skied late summer day, the kind that gives my face a constant sheen and makes Helena's hair curl.

"Mama, can we cross?" Helena says. She has left the pavement of the wide walk and is standing on the grass that slopes to a small creek.

"Yeah, but keep to the rocks," I say and go closer.

She edges down the grass watching her feet. She stops in the gravel of the creek's edge and stands with her shoulders back and one foot propped on a rock the size of a loaf of bread. She waits. She looks like Michelangelo's *David*.

I walk to her. Her little back is strong. Her face is away from me and might be watching the water curl around the rocks or planning where she will put her feet. The ends of her fingers twitch.

"Mama," she says and turns around.

I'm not Mama Bear anymore, but I can't tell you when it happened.

"Yes," I say.

"Come here," Helena says and she waves her hand in a circle by her face.

I kneel down and my toes push into the gravel.

"I have to tell you something," Helena says. Our heads are level and she puts her hands on my cheeks. She is smiling, and her face is close to mine.

"What is it?" I say.

"I have to tell you a secret," she says. She turns my head and brings it to the side of hers so our ears touch and our cheeks touch, and we are both looking now to the other side of the creek. Someday she'll tell a secret like the rest of us, with her hand cupped around her mouth as she leans into an ear, but I want to remember the way she is doing it now. I love how she is doing it now. One of Helena's hands is still on my face. Her hair brushes my ear.

"It tickles," I say and laugh and pull away to scratch.

"No, Mama," she says. "Come back; I have to tell you something. It's a secret."

"Oh, a secret! Why didn't you say so?"

"I did say so!" she says and waves her hand again. "Come here."

I lean in. She pulls my face next to hers again until our cheeks are pressed together.

"I love you," I whisper.

"The secret!"

"Yes, the secret."

Her cheek is cool.

I hear a bird.

She whispers into the open space in front us.

afterword

When I was about a year into trying to have a second child, I ran into a friend from high school who asked me if Chad and I were "planning on having a second." I told him yes, that we had been trying, but that it wasn't happening. He squinched his face and looked over my shoulder and said, "Really? That's weird. I've heard of people having trouble with their first, but the second always seems to happen easily."

I had heard those stories, too. My impression was that the overwhelming majority of people having trouble with infertility were people who couldn't get pregnant at all. In fact, when I went to the bookstore one morning, harried and desperate, I picked up book after book about women who did not have any children and who were trying anything to get one. I felt guilty (how audacious of me to be feeling desperate and sorry for myself for not being able to have two!). But then I also felt more alone. Maybe it really is weird to experience difficulty having a second child. And with this thought I developed split thinking: You are either an infertile person or you are not. And since I had Helena, I was obviously not. Looking back, it's really crazy how often I thought, *But I have Helena; what would have changed?* as if in having one child I was forever exempt from infertility. Even though I knew infertility was a designation defined by length of trying with no results, I still felt like it didn't apply to me.

So here's the really embarrassing part: Despite eventually finding out about other women experiencing difficulties, despite my gynecologist suggesting Clomid, despite so much time passing, it wasn't until finishing this book that I actually went online, did some research and found out about secondary infertility. I never even knew there was a term that defined my situation. And what blew me away about it, and what I wished I had known all along, is how prevalent the problem seems to be. Apparently struggling to have a second child isn't strange at all. I don't know if knowing that years ago would have changed any of my actions, but it would have at least put a stop to the thought *I have Helena; what could have changed.* And while I can get pretty fired up about feeling like one of my doctors should have told me about this, I also realize that three years ago I could have spent two hours on Google like I did three months ago and I would have found it. It's just that I wasn't looking.

bibliography

Dickinson, Emily. "254." *The Poems of Emily Dickinson*. Ed. Thomas H. Johnson. Cambridge, Massachusetts: The Belknap Press of Harvard University Press, 1951.

Melville, Herman. *Moby Dick*. 1851. Introd. Alfred Kazin. Boston: Riverside-Houghton, 1956.

Made in the USA
Lexington, KY
20 April 2016